Imaging Atlas of
Human
Anatomy
Second Edition

Jamie Weir
MB BS DMRD FRCP(Ed) FRCR
Clinical Professor of Radiology
Aberdeen Royal Hospitals NHS Trust
Aberdeen, UK

Peter H Abrahams
MB BS FRCS(Ed) FRCR
Fellow of Girton College, Cambridge, UK
Professor of Clinical Anatomy
Kigezi International School of Medicine
Cambridge Overseas Programme
Family Practitioner, London, UK

with five contributors

Margaret D Hourihan
MB BCh FRCR
Consultant Neuroradiologist
Department of Radiology
University Hospital of Wales
Cardiff, UK

Anna-Maria Belli
MB BS DMRD FRCR
Consultant Radiologist and Honorary Senior Lecturer
Department of Diagnostic Radiology
St George's Hospital
London, UK

Niall R Moore
MA MB BChir MRCP FRCR
Lecturer and Honorary Consultant Radiologist
Department of Radiology
University of Oxford
Oxford, UK

Gillian Needham
BSc MB ChB FRCR
Consultant Radiologist
Aberdeen Royal Hospitals NHS Trust
Aberdeen, UK

J Philip Owen
MB BS DMRD FRCR
Senior Lecturer and Honorary Consultant Radiologist
Department of Radiology
University of Newcastle upon Tyne
Newcastle upon Tyne, UK

 Mosby

London   Philadelphia   St Louis   Sydney   Tokyo

ISBN   0 7234 2283 4

Copyright © 1997 Times Mirror International Publishers Limited.

Published in 1997 by Mosby-Wolfe, an imprint of Times Mirror International Publishers Limited.

Reprinted in 1998 by Mosby, an imprint of Mosby International.

Image reproduction and final film by Spectrum Colour, Ipswich, UK.

Printed and bound by Vincenzo Bona s.r.l., Turin, Italy.

For full details of all Mosby titles, please write to Mosby, Lynton House, 7–12 Tavistock Square, London WC1H 9LB, UK.

A CIP catalogue record for this book is available from the British Library and the US Library of Congress.

Project Manager	Sarah Gray
Development Editor	Simon Pritchard
Designer	Ian Spick
Illustration	Mike Saiz
Layout	Gisli Thor, Paul Wilkinson
Index	Anita Reid
Production	Siobhan Egan
Publisher	Geoff Greenwood

Contents

Acknowledgements

We are indebted to the following for lending us images for publication:

Professor D J Allison, Hammersmith Hospital, London, UK (page 137,B and page 140,B)

Dr A Clifton, Atkinson Morley's Hospital, London, UK (page 64, B)

Dr J Jackson, Hammersmith Hospital, London, UK (page 140, A)

Dr I W McCall, Robert Jones and Agnes Hunt Hospital, Oswestry, UK (page 64, A)

Miss Elaine Sassoon, Department of Plastic Surgery, University College London, London, UK (page 20, B)

The following have kindly lent us new images for the second edition:

Dr R Clements, Royal Gwent Hospital, Newport, UK (prostatic ultrasound)

Dr P A Dubbins, Derriford Hospital, Plymouth, UK (general abdominal and pelvic ultrasound)

Dr A Rickards, The Middlesex Hospital, London, UK (penile arteriogram and IV cavernosogram)

Dr S A Russell, St Mary's Hospital, Manchester, UK (fetal ultrasound and neonatal cranial ultrasound)

We are also indebted to Drs Philip Bearcroft, Nick Screaton, Maneesh Patel, Hilary Moss, Charlie Hardingham, Russell Bull and Jonathan Gillard for their diligent checking of page proofs.

Preface

In the four years since the production of the first edition of *An Imaging Atlas of Human Anatomy*, imaging has improved considerably, particularly in the fields of magnetic resonance and ultrasound. Over half the images have been updated for this new edition. Further improvements include the addition of completely new sections, limb ossification dates, line diagrams to improve the understanding of difficult areas and increased numbers of views where appropriate.

Most of the magnetic resonance images have been replaced with improved image recording, leading to greater clarity of anatomical detail. Ultrasound images have been similarly changed to be more comprehensive and cohesive. Examples of magnetic resonance angiography are included not only to demonstrate the remarkable beauty of these images but also to show the future of angiography into the next millennium.

It is with regret that one of our original authors, Professor Anne Hemingway, has left the team, but our thanks go to her for all her help and encouragement. We have pestered more outside contributors, as is evident from the list of acknowledgements, and our thanks go to them for their images and specialist expertise.

The CD-ROM version of our first edition was successfully launched late in 1995. The multimedia platform offers real-time ultrasound sequences, self-testing features and fully interactive labelling. Version 2.0 of the CD-ROM will be launched alongside this new edition of the book.

Imaging has opened up further anatomical areas to study and will continue to do so. We hope this new edition will stimulate its readers to explore the body through imaging as a key to its understanding.

Jamie Weir, Peter Abrahams
September 1996

Preface to the first edition

Imaging methods used to display normal human anatomy have improved dramatically over the last few decades. The ability to demonstrate the soft tissues by using the modern technologies of magnetic resonance imaging, X-ray computed tomography, and ultrasound has greatly facilitated our understanding of the link between anatomy as shown in the dissecting room and that necessary for clinical practice. This Atlas has been produced because of the new technology and the fundamental changes that are occurring in the teaching of anatomy. It enables the preclinical medical student to relate to basic anatomy while, at the same time, providing a comprehensive study guide for the clinical interpretation of imaging, applicable for all undergraduate and postgraduate levels.

Several distinguished authors, experts in their own fields of imaging, have contributed to this book, which has benefited from editorial integration to ensure balance and cohesion. The Atlas is designed to complement and supplement the *Colour Atlas of Human Anatomy* by McMinn.

Duplication of images occurs only where it is necessary to demonstrate anatomical points of interest or difficulty. Similarly, examples of different imaging modalities of the same anatomical region are only included if they contribute to a better understanding of the region shown. Radiographs that show important landmarks in limb ossification centre development, together with examples of some common congenital anomalies, are also documented. In certain sections, notably MR and CT, the legends may cover more than one page, so that a specific structure can be followed in continuity through various levels and planes.

Human anatomy does not alter, but our methods of demonstrating it have changed significantly. Modern imaging allows certain structures and their relationships to be seen for the first time, and this has aided us in their interpretation. Knowledge and understanding of radiological anatomy are fundamental to all those involved in patient care, from the nurse and the paramedic to medical students and clinicians.

Jamie Weir, Peter Abrahams
February 1992

To our students,

past, present and future

Guide to ossification tables

Ossification tables, such as the one shown on the right, appear throughout this book.

The key to these tables is as follows:
(c) = cartilage
(m) = membrane
miu = months of intrauterine life
wiu = weeks of intrauterine life
mths = months
yrs = years

And the rule to remember is: girls before boys.

CLAVICLE (m)	Appears	Fused
Lateral end	5 wiu	20+ yrs
Medial end	15 yrs	20+ yrs
SCAPULA (c)		
Body	8 wiu	15 yrs
Coracoid	<1 yr	20 yrs
Coracoid base	Puberty	15–20 yrs
Acromion	Puberty	15–20 yrs

Introduction

Angiography

Access to the arterial system in order to produce an arteriogram (angiogram) is usually obtained by puncture and catheterisation of a femoral artery under local anaesthesia. Radiographic contrast medium is then injected into the vessel in the area under examination. If, for some reason, access via the femoral artery is not possible (owing to iliac occlusive disease or the presence of a graft, for example), alternative sites, such as the brachial or axillary artery, can be used. Translumbar aortography (TLA), a method of arteriography that involves direct percutaneous puncture of the aorta, is now less commonly employed as it does not allow selective catheterisation of aortic branches and hence percutaneous interventional vascular procedures cannot be performed. The development of new technology has meant that the aorta and the main upper and lower limb arteries can be visualised from an intravenous injection of contrast medium (into brachial vein, superior vena cava or right atrium), obviating the need for arterial puncture in some patients. This technique employs digital subtraction angiography (DSA), whereby unwanted background information is 'subtracted', leaving only an image of the blood vessels. Images of arteries obtained by injection into a vein are referred to as intravenous DSA examinations (IV DSA). DSA images of arteries can, of course, be obtained by direct intra-arterial injection (IA DSA).

Manual photographic subtraction of background information can also be performed with conventional (nondigital) arteriography. Subtraction, either photographic or digital, is used in cases in which fine vascular detail is required and can be simply recognised by the fact that, in contrast to an unsubtracted film, the arteries appear black as opposed to white. Different radiographic projections are sometimes employed to visualise best the vasculature; for example, in the aortic arch an anteroposterior view may not clearly show the origins of the vessels arising from the arch as they are very close to each other and may be superimposed. A left anterior oblique position opens the arch, allowing better visualisation of the origins of the brachiocephalic, left carotid and subclavian arteries. The angiograms in this book use the anteroposterior (AP) projection, unless otherwise indicated.

Veins may be visualised in the same way as the arteries, by direct puncture and catheterisation (via the femoral vein in most instances), for example. The veins of the upper and lower limbs are imaged by injecting contrast medium via an 18G or 20G needle placed in a peripheral vein, such as in the dorsum of the foot or hand, or the antecubital fossa. Alternatively, if imaging from an arterial injection is continued over a prolonged period of time, the arterial, capillary and venous phases can be recorded and venous anatomy visualised; this is a particularly useful way of visualising the portal venous system without necessitating direct trans-splenic or transhepatic puncture.

Specialist texts should be consulted for details of arterial puncture, catheterisation and imaging techniques and for information on the type of equipment used in angiography.

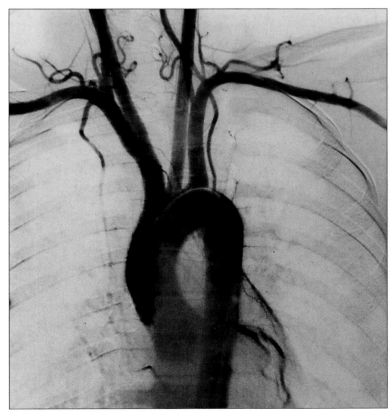

Subtracted arch aortogram (page 111, A).

Renal arteriogram (page 139, A).

Computed tomography

The limitation of all plain radiographic techniques is their two-dimensional representation of three-dimensional structures: the linear attenuation coefficients of all of the tissues in the path of the X-ray beam form the image.

Computed tomography (CT) obtains a series of different angular X-ray projections that are processed by a computer to give a section of specified thickness. The CT image comprises a regular matrix of picture elements (pixels). All of the tissues contained within the pixel attenuate the X-ray projections and result in a mean attenuation value for the pixel. This value is compared with the attenuation value of water and is displayed on a scale (the Hounsfield scale). Water is said to have an attenuation of 0 Hounsfield units (HU), and the scale is 2000 HU wide. Air typically has an HU number of −1000; fat is approximately −100 HU; soft tissues are in the range +20 to +70 HU; and bone is greater than +400 HU.

The CT machine consists of a rigid metal frame with an X-ray tube sited opposite a set of detectors. In early designs the tube and detectors scanned across the patient and then rotated to a different position ('translate–rotate'). Current third-generation CT machines have a wider detector array and an X-ray fan beam, which encompasses the whole patient. All the views per slice can be collected simultaneously so that the tube and detectors only rotate around the patient. Routine acquisition times are 2–4 seconds, although a variant of the design utilises a constantly rotating tube–detector system that results in subsecond scan times.

All CT machines, of whatever generation, share similar components. The detectors are either gas ionisation chambers or scintillation crystals linked to photomultiplier tubes. The signal is digitised by an analogue-to-digital converter (ADC) in the gantry. The digitised signal is transferred to the image processing computer and subsequently displayed on the operator's console. Images are usually photographed on medical recording film (hard copy) using optical or laser cameras. For long-term storage, the data set is transferred to magnetic media (tape or disc) or to optical disc.

No specific preparation is required for examinations of the brain, spine, musculoskeletal system and chest. Studies of the abdomen and pelvis almost always require opacification of gastrointestinal tract, using a solution of dilute contrast medium (either water-soluble or a barium compound). Generally, 750–1000 ml are given orally 30–60 minutes prior to imaging, with the final 300 ml taken as the patient enters the examination room. The large bowel may also be opacified using a solution of contrast medium administered rectally, either in a preparation room or on the CT table. Examinations of the female pelvis are often performed after the insertion of a vaginal tampon to facilitate interpretation.

Identification of vascular structures may be made on the basis of anatomy alone, but the intravenous injection of water-soluble contrast medium may be required. Techniques vary according to the individual case, but the most common method is to inject a bolus of 50 ml followed by a rapid infusion of 50 ml, using contrast medium containing 300–370 mg iodine/ml.

Generally, all studies are performed with the patient supine, and images are obtained in the transverse plane. Modern CT machines allow up to 25° of gantry angulation, which is particularly valuable in spinal imaging. Occasionally, coronal images are obtained in the investigation of cranial abnormalities; in these cases the patient lies prone, with the neck extended, and the gantry is angled appropriately.

Lungs (left, page 99, N) and male pelvis (right, page 148, C), axial CT images.

Magnetic resonance imaging

Magnetic resonance imaging (MRI) combines a strong magnetic field and radiofrequency (RF) energy to study the distribution and behaviour of hydrogen protons in fat and water.

The spinning proton of the hydrogen nucleus can be thought of as a tiny bar magnet, with a north and south pole. In the absence of an external magnetic field, the magnetic moments of all of the protons in the body are randomly arranged. However, when the patient is placed in a strong magnetic field these magnetic moments align either with or against the field lines of the magnet. A small excess of magnetic moments align with the field, so that a net magnetic vector is established.

RF energy is used to generate a second magnetic field, perpendicular to the static magnetic field of the machine. The result of this second magnetic field is to rotate or 'flip' the protons away from the static magnetic field; the amount of rotation depends on the quantity of RF energy absorbed. Once the RF field is switched off, the protons experience only the effects of the static magnetic field and flip back to their original position. During this return to equilibrium, a process called 'relaxation', protons emit the RF energy they had acquired. This energy is detected by the antenna in the MRI machine, digitised, amplified and, finally, spatially encoded by the array processor. The resulting images are displayed on the operator's console and can be recorded on hard copy (for viewing) or transferred to magnetic tape or optical disc (for storage).

MRI systems are graded according to the strength of the magnetic field they produce. High-field systems are those capable of producing a magnetic field strength of 1–2 Tesla (T; 10 000–20 000 Gauss); mid-field systems operate at 0.35–0.5 T; and low-field systems produce a field strength of less than 0.2 T. Mid- and high-field systems use superconducting magnets in which the coils of copper wire are kept in a superconducting state (−269°C) by being immersed in an insulated helium bath. Electromagnets are fitted in resistive systems and are limited by heating factors to 0.35 T. Low-field systems use permanently magnetised metal cores, limiting field strength to around 0.2 T.

MRI does not present any recognised biological hazard. Patients who have any form of pacemaker or implanted electro-inductive device must not be examined. Other prohibited items include ferromagnetic intracranial aneurysm slips, certain types of cardiac valve replacement and intra-ocular metallic foreign bodies. Generally, it is safe to examine patients who have extracranial vascular clips and orthopaedic prostheses, but these may cause local artefacts. Loose metal items must be excluded from the examination room.

The preparation for an MR examination is simple. Patients wear metal-free clothes and must answer a rigorous safety questionnaire. Antiperistaltic agents (e.g. parenteral hyoscine N-butylbromide or glucagon) are often used in abdominal and pelvic examinations. Software techniques counteract respiratory motion for chest and abdominal imaging. Electrocardiographic gating is used in cardiac studies.

MR images may be obtained in any orthogonal or non-orthogonal plane. There is a wide range of pulse sequences, each of which provides a different image contrast. An intravenous injection of contrast medium (a gadolinium complex) may be given to enhance the visualisation of tumours, and inflammatory and vascular abnormalities.

Magnetic resonance angiography

The appearance of blood vessels depends on the pulse sequence used to produce images. With the spin echo technique, the time that elapses between exciting protons and receiving the return signal (the echo time) is such that excited blood has flowed out of the region; this volume of blood is replaced by unexcited blood which does not produce a signal, resulting in a flow void.

Gradient echo sequences use short echo-collection times and more frequent RF excitations, so that protons in stationary tissues do not fully relax, reducing the signal they generate. Protons entering the slice, however, are fully relaxed and thus produce a high signal (the 'time of flight effect'), so that blood vessels appear as bright structures against a dark background. Images can be displayed as three-dimensional MR angiograms, which can be viewed from any angle.

Another MR angiography technique uses additional magnetic fields to encode the phase of moving protons in blood vessels. A complete assessment of flow requires three acquisitions, each encoded by one of the three orthogonal gradients. These are summed to produce a 'phase contrast' MR angiogram. Phase differences can be quantified to provide estimates of flow velocity.

Brain, axial MR image
(page 42, B).

Arteries of the brain, axial
MRA (page 32, A).

Ultrasound

In contrast with the other images in this book, ultrasound images do not depend on the use of electromagnetic wave forms. It is the properties of high-frequency sound waves (longitudinal waves) and their interaction with biological tissues that go to form these 'echograms'.

A sound wave of appropriate frequency (diagnostic range 3.5–10 MHz) is produced by piezo-electric principles. Both the size and shape of the emitting crystal and its resonant frequency are important factors in determining the course of the sound beam within the tissues to be examined.

As the beam passes through tissues, two important effects determine image production: attenuation and reflection. Attenuation is caused by the loss of energy from the system, due to absorption and reflection, refraction and beam divergence out of the range of the receiver. The greater the attenuation of the sound beam through the tissues, the lower the resultant signal intensity received. Reflection of sound waves within the range of the receiver produces the image, the texture of which is dependent upon differences in acoustic impedance between different tissues. Ultrasound imaging systems are sensitive to the very small changes in acoustic impedance within soft tissue.

Through the application of these basic principles, sophisticated hardware has been developed that converts the pulse–echo system, briefly described above, into a real-time two-dimensional sectional image. The addition of the facility to measure blood flow and velocity ultrasonically (using the Doppler principle) has led to the development and wide availability of duplex scanners.

The effects of shadowing and enhancement within an ultrasound image are of paramount importance. Systems are designed assuming an average attenuation through a depth of tissue, and are balanced to give an even intensity of signal for deep and superficial tissues. An acoustic shadow occurs when a tissue within the measured depth has a higher-than-average attenuation; all tissues deep to this will appear with a falsely lower intensity (shadowed). Conversely, a tissue with a lower-than-average attenuation will cause all tissues deep to it to appear falsely high in intensity (enhanced). Fibrous tissue, calcification and gas all produce acoustic shadows, whereas fluid-filled structures often cause enhancement.

If a selection of ultrasound transducers with varying frequencies, focusing mechanisms and shapes and sizes is available, visualisation of a wide range of tissues—from the neonatal brain to the soft tissues of the hand—becomes possible. Only relevant ultrasound images have been included in the book to illustrate a particular point or area, as the real-time nature of ultrasound precludes further coverage. Interpretation of the anatomy from static ultrasound images is more difficult than that from other imaging modalities because the technique is highly operator-dependent and provides information on tissue structure and form different from that of other imaging techniques.

Neonatal brain (page 42, A), ultrasound image.

Abdomen (page 130, D), ultrasound image.

Head, neck and brain

(a) Skull, occipitofrontal projection.
(b) Skull, demonstrating the foramina rotunda, occipitofrontal projection.

1 Basi-occiput
2 Body of sphenoid
3 Crista galli
4 Ethmoidal air cells
5 Floor of maxillary sinus (antrum)
6 Foramen rotundum
7 Frontal sinus
8 Greater wing of sphenoid
9 Internal acoustic meatus
10 Lambdoid suture
11 Lateral mass of atlas (first cervical vertebra)
12 Lesser wing of sphenoid
13 Mastoid process
14 Nasal septum
15 Odontoid process (dens) of axis (second cervical vertebra)
16 Petrous part of temporal bone
17 Sagittal suture
18 Sella turcica
19 Superior orbital fissure
20 Temporal surface of greater wing of sphenoid

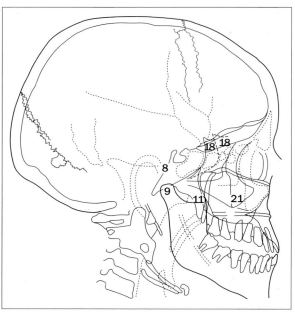

(a) Skull, lateral projection.

Pituitary fossa (sella turcica), (b) of a 7-year-old child, (c) of a 23-year-old woman, lateral projections.

1	Anterior arch of atlas (first cervical vertebra)	11	Coronoid process of mandible	22	Mastoid air cells
2	Anterior clinoid process	12	Diploë	23	Middle clinoid process
3	Arch of zygoma	13	Dorsum sellae	24	Odontoid process (dens) of axis (second
4	Articular tubercle for temporomandibular	14	Ethmoidal air cells		cervical vertebra)
	joint	15	External acoustic meatus	25	Palatine process of maxilla
5	Basilar part of occipital bone	16	Frontal process of zygoma	26	Pituitary fossa (sella turcica)
6	Basisphenoid/basi-occiput synchondrosis	17	Frontal sinus	27	Planum sphenoidale
7	Carotid sulcus	18	Greater wing of sphenoid	28	Posterior clinoid process
8	Clivus	19	Grooves for middle meningeal vessels	29	Ramus of mandible
9	Condyle of mandible	20	Lambdoid suture	30	Sphenoidal sinus
10	Coronal suture	21	Malar process of maxilla	31	Tuberculum sellae

Skull, 30º fronto-occipital (Townes') projection.

1 Arch of atlas (first cervical vertebra)
2 Arcuate eminence of temporal bone
3 Coronal suture
4 Dorsum sellae
5 Foramen magnum
6 Internal acoustic meatus
7 Lambdoid suture
8 Mandibular condyle
9 Odontoid process (dens) of axis (second cervical vertebra)
10 Sagittal suture
11 Superior semicircular canal
12 Zygomatic arch

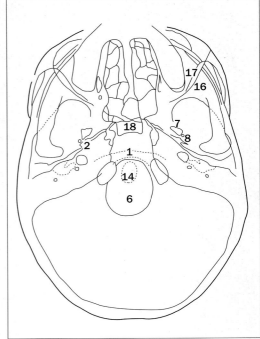

(a) Skull, submentovertical projection.
(b) Skull, with additional angulation for zygomatic arches, submentovertical projection.

1	Anterior arch of atlas (first cervical vertebra)
2	Auditory (Eustachian) tube
3	Body of mandible
4	Carotid canal
5	Foramen lacerum
6	Foramen magnum
7	Foramen ovale
8	Foramen spinosum
9	Greater palatine foramen
10	Greater wing of sphenoid
11	Head of mandible
12	Jugular foramen
13	Occipital condyle
14	Odontoid process (dens) of axis (second cervical vertebra)
15	Perpendicular plate of ethmoid
16	Posterior margin of orbit
17	Posterior wall of maxillary sinus (antrum)
18	Sphenoidal sinus
19	Temporal process of zygomatic bone
20	Vomer
21	Zygomatic arch
22	Zygomatic bone
23	Zygomatic process of temporal bone

Facial bones and paranasal sinuses, **(a)** occipitofrontal projection, **(b)** occipitomental projection, **(c)** lateral projection.

1 Anterior wall of maxillary sinus (antrum)
2 Condyle of mandible
3 Coronoid process of mandible
4 Ethmoidal sinuses
5 Frontal process of zygomatic bone
6 Frontal sinuses
7 Frontozygomatic suture
8 Greater wing of sphenoid
9 Horizontal plate of palatine bone
10 Infra-orbital foramen
11 Left maxillary sinus (antrum)
12 Lesser wing of sphenoid
13 Malar process of maxilla
14 Nasal septum
15 Palatine process of maxilla
16 Posterior wall of maxillary sinus (antrum)
17 Sella turcica
18 Sphenoidal sinus
19 Superior orbital fissure
20 Temporal process of zygomatic bone
21 Zygomatic arch
22 Zygomatic process of frontal bone
23 Zygomatic process of temporal bone

Facial bones and paranasal sinuses, axial CT images are demonstrated at the following levels: **(a)** hard palate; **(b)** inferior nasal turbinate; **(c)** maxillary sinus; **(d)** middle turbinates; **(e)** ethmoidal sinuses; **(f)** ethmoidal sinuses and upper sphenoidal sinus; **(g)** optic nerve; **(h)** frontal sinus.

1 Alveolar recess	**12** Foramen ovale	**24** Inferolateral recess
2 Alveolar rim	**13** Foramen spinosum	**25** Infratemporal fossa
3 Anterior arch of atlas (first cervical vertebra)	**14** Frontal bone	**26** Internal acoustic meatus
	15 Frontal sinus	**27** Lacrimal bone
4 Anterior clinoid process	**16** Globe	**28** Lateral pterygoid muscle
5 Anterior ethmoidal air cells	**17** Greater palatine canal	**29** Lateral pterygoid plate
6 Clivus	**18** Greater wing of sphenoid	**30** Lateral wall of maxillary sinus (antrum)
7 Coronoid process of mandible	**19** Hard palate	**31** Lens
8 Crista galli	**20** Head of mandible	**32** Mandibular condyle
9 Deglutitional muscles	**21** Incisive canal	**33** Masseter muscle
10 Dorsum sellae	**22** Inferior nasal concha (turbinate)	**34** Mastoid air cells
11 External acoustic canal	**23** Inferior orbital fissure	**35** Mastoid process

36 Maxillary sinus (antrum)	**47** Nasopharynx	**58** Sphenoidal sinus
37 Medial pterygoid muscle	**48** Odontoid process (dens)	**59** Spinal canal
38 Medial pterygoid plate	**49** Optic canal	**60** Styloid process
39 Medial wall of maxillary sinus (antrum)	**50** Optic nerve	**61** Superior orbital fissure
40 Middle concha (turbinate)	**51** Oropharynx	**62** Temporal lobe
41 Middle cranial fossa	**52** Parapharyngeal space	**63** Temporalis muscle
42 Middle ear cavity	**53** Perpendicular plate of ethmoid bone	**64** Vomer
43 Middle ethmoidal air cells	**54** Posterior ethmoidal air cells	**65** Zygoma
44 Nasal bone	**55** Pterygoid fossa	**66** Zygomatic arch
45 Nasal cavity	**56** Pterygomaxillary fissure	
46 Nasolacrimal duct	**57** Ramus of mandible	

Facial bones and paranasal sinuses, coronal CT images are demonstrated at the following levels: **(a)** frontal sinus; **(b)** anterior maxillary sinus and ethmoidal sinuses; **(c)** middle ethmoidal sinus and maxillary sinus; **(d)** middle maxillary sinus; **(e)** posterior ethmoidal sinus; **(f)** posterior maxillary sinus; **(g)** anterior sphenoidal sinus; **(h)** posterior sphenoidal sinus.

1	Alveolar rim	**11**	Frontal bone
2	Anterior clinoid process	**12**	Frontal sinus
3	Anterior ethmoidal air cells	**13**	Frontozygomatic suture
4	Cartilaginous portion of nasal septum	**14**	Globe
5	Cribriform plate	**15**	Greater wing of sphenoid
6	Crista galli	**16**	Hard palate
7	Diploe	**17**	Inferior nasal concha (turbinate)
8	Dorsum sellae	**18**	Inferior orbital fissure
9	Foramen lacerum	**19**	Infra-orbital canal
10	Foramen ovale	**20**	Infratemporal fossa

21 Lamina papyracea	**32** Perpendicular plate of ethmoidal bone
22 Lesser wing of sphenoid	**33** Planum sphenoidale
23 Maxillary sinus (antrum)	**34** Posterior ethmoidal air cells
24 Middle concha (turbinate)	**35** Pterygopalatine fossa
25 Middle ethmoidal air cells	**36** Ramus of mandible
26 Middle meatus	**37** Sphenoidal sinus
27 Nasal bone	**38** Superior orbital fissure
28 Nasolacrimal duct	**39** Temporal lobe
29 Nasopharynx	**40** Vomer
30 Optic canal	**41** Zygoma
31 Ostium of antrum	

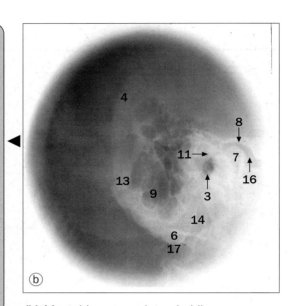

1 Aditus to mastoid antrum
2 Arcuate eminence of temporal bone
3 External acoustic meatus
4 Helix of pinna of ear
5 Internal acoustic meatus
6 Lateral sinus
7 Mandibular condyle
8 Mandibular fossa
9 Mastoid air cells
10 Orbital margin
11 Ossicles (malleus, incus)
12 Petrous part of temporal bone
13 Pinna of ear
14 Styloid process
15 Superior semicircular canal
16 Temporomandibular joint
17 Tip of mastoid process
18 Vestibular part of inner ear
19 Zygomatic arch

(a) Petrous temporal bone, postero-anterior oblique projection.

(b) Mastoid process, lateral oblique projection.

Temporomandibular joint, sagittal MR images, (c) closed, (d) open.
Radiographs of the temporomandibular joint, (e) closed, (f) open.

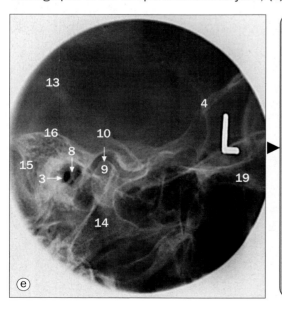

1 Articular disc
2 Articular tubercle of temporal bone
3 External acoustic meatus
4 Greater wing of sphenoid
5 Head of mandible
6 Inferior temporal gyrus
7 Lateral pterygoid muscle
8 Malleus
9 Mandibular condyle
10 Mandibular fossa
11 Mastoid process of temporal bone
12 Neck of mandible
13 Pinna of ear
14 Posterior border of ramus of mandible
15 Sinus plate
16 Tegmen tympani
17 Transverse sinus
18 Tympanic part of temporal bone
19 Zygomatic process of temporal bone

(a) Temporal bone, tomogram at level of internal acoustic meatus.

1	Carotid canal	7	Mastoid antrum
2	Cochlea	8	Petrous part of temporal
3	External acoustic meatus		bone
4	Incus	9	Styloid process of temporal
5	Internal acoustic meatus		bone
6	Malleus	10	Superior semicircular canal

(b) Temporal bone, tomogram at level of cochlea (image taken several millimetres anterior to section shown in (a)).

(c) Temporal bone, CT image.
(d) Temporal bone, axial MR image through cerebellopontine angle.

1	Abducens nerve	10	Geniculate ganglion	19	Mastoid air cells
2	Aditus ad antrum	11	Incudomalleolar joint	20	Pons
3	Aerated petrous apex	12	Incus	21	Posterior semicircular canal
4	Basilar artery in prepontine cistern	13	Inferior petrosal sinus	22	Scutum
5	Cerebellar hemisphere	14	Internal acoustic canal	23	Sphenoidal sinus
6	Cochlea	15	Internal occipital protuberance	24	Superior orbital fissure
7	Epitympanum	16	Lambdoid suture	25	Temporal lobe
8	Facial nerve	17	Lateral semicircular canal	26	Vestibule
9	Facial nerve (first part)	18	Malleus	27	Vestibulocochlear nerve

Temporal bones, axial CT images are demonstrated at the following levels: (a) external acoustic canal; (b) cochlea; (c) internal acoustic canal and vestibule; (d) upper middle ear and mastoid.

1 Aditus to antrum	**12** Dorsum sellae	**23** Greater wing of sphenoid
2 Aeration of petrous apex	**13** Epitympanic space	**24** Horizontal portion of canal for facial nerve
3 Atlanto-occipital joint	**14** Ethmoidal air cells	**25** Hypoglossal canal
4 Auditory (Eustachian) tube	**15** External acoustic canal	**26** Incudomalleolar joint
5 Brainstem	**16** External acoustic meatus	**27** Incus
6 Carotid canal	**17** Facial nerve (first part)	**28** Internal acoustic canal
7 Cerebellum	**18** Facial recess	**29** Internal acoustic meatus
8 Clivus	**19** Falciform crest	**30** Internal occipital protuberance
9 Cochlea	**20** Foramen ovale	**31** Jugular foramen
10 Cochlear aqueduct	**21** Geniculate ganglion	**32** Jugular fossa
11 Descending segment of facial nerve	**22** Greater petrosal nerve	**33** Jugular tubercle

Temporal bones, coronal CT images are demonstrated at the following levels:
(e) posterior temporomandibular joint; **(f)** external acoustic meatus and vestibule; **(g)** internal acoustic meatus; **(h)** mastoid.

34 Lambdoid suture	**45** Oval window	**57** Stylomastoid foramen
35 Lateral mass of atlas (first cervical vertebra)	**46** Petro-occipital fissure	**58** Sulcus of sigmoid venous sinus
	47 Petrous temporal bone	**59** Superior orbital fissure
36 Lateral semicircular canal	**48** Pinna of ear	**60** Superior semicircular canal
37 Malleus	**49** Posterior semicircular canal	**61** Tegmen tympani
38 Mastoid air cells	**50** Pyramidal eminence	**62** Temporal lobe
39 Mastoid antrum	**51** Scutum	**63** Temporomandibular joint
40 Middle ear cavity	**52** Sinus tympani	**64** Tensor tympani muscle
41 Nasopharynx	**53** Sphenoidal sinus	**65** Tip of mastoid process
42 Occipital bone	**54** Squamous temporal bone	**66** Vestibular aqueduct
43 Occipital condyle	**55** Stapes	**67** Vestibule
44 Odontoid process (dens)	**56** Styloid process	

(a) and (b) Skull base, axial CT images.

1	Articular condyle	12	Foramen ovale	23	Occipital bone
2	Auditory (Eustachian) tube	13	Foramen spinosum	24	Petro-occipital fissure
3	Basisphenoid	14	Globe	25	Pinna of ear
4	Caroticojugular spine	15	Greater wing of sphenoid	26	Pterygoid (vidian) canal
5	Carotid canal	16	Inferior orbital fissure	27	Pterygomaxillary fissure
6	Cerebellar hemisphere	17	Jugular foramen	28	Pterygopalantine fossa
7	Clivus	18	Lens	29	Sphenoidal sinus
8	Ethmoidal air cells	19	Mandibular condyle	30	Sulcus of sigmoid venous sinus
9	External acoustic meatus	20	Mandibular fossa	31	Temporalis muscle
10	Facial nerve canal	21	Mastoid air cells		
11	Foramen lacerum	22	Nasal septum		

(c) and (d) Skull base, coronal CT images.

1	Atlanto-axial joint	7	Jugular fossa	13	Pinna of ear
2	Atlanto-occipital joint	8	Jugular tubercle	14	Posterior fossa
3	Axis (second cervical vertebra)	9	Lateral mass of atlas (first cervical vertebra)	15	Styloid process
4	Cerebral hemisphere	10	Mastoid air cells	16	Stylomastoid foramen
5	Descending segment of canal for facial nerve	11	Occipital condyle	17	Tentorium cerebelli
6	Hypoglossal canal	12	Odontoid process (dens)	18	Transverse process of atlas

(a) Orbital venogram. ▲

1	Angular veins
2	Anterior collateral vein
3	Cavernous sinus
4	First part of superior ophthalmic vein
5	Frontal veins
6	Inferior ophthalmic vein
7	Internal carotid artery
8	Medial collateral vein
9	Second part of superior ophthalmic vein
10	Superficial connecting vein
11	Supraorbital vein
12	Third part of superior ophthalmic vein

(b) Macrodacryocystogram. ▲

1	Common canaliculus	**5**	Lacrimal sac
2	Hard palate	**6**	Nasolacrimal duct
3	Inferior canaliculus	**7**	Site of lacrimal punctum
4	Lacrimal catheters	**8**	Superior canaliculus

(c) Globe, axial MR image.

1	Anterior chamber	**10**	Optic nerve
2	Aqueous humour	**11**	Retina and choroid
3	Cornea	**12**	Retro-orbital fat
4	Ethmoidal sinuses	**13**	Sclera
5	Eyelid	**14**	Suspensory ligament of the lens
6	Lateral rectus muscle		
7	Lens	**15**	Temporalis muscle
8	Medial rectus muscle	**16**	Vitreous
9	Ophthalmic artery		

(a)–(h) Nasopharynx and oropharynx, axial MR images.

1 Alveolar process of maxilla	**8** Body of mandible	**16** Fat in infratemporal fossa	**25** Internal carotid artery
2 Anterior arch of atlas (first cervical vertebra)	**9** Buccinator muscle	**17** Fourth ventricle	**26** Internal jugular vein
3 Anterior facial vein	**10** Cerebellar tonsils	**18** Genioglossus muscle	**27** Intrinsic muscles of tongue
4 Ascending pharyngeal artery	**11** Cerebrospinal fluid in subarachnoid space	**19** Hard palate	**28** Lateral mass of atlas (first cervical vertebra)
5 Auditory (Eustachian) tube	**12** Coronoid process of mandible	**20** Head of mandible	**29** Lateral pharyngeal recess
6 Basilar artery	**13** Deep lobe of parotid gland	**21** Hyoglossus muscle	**30** Lateral pterygoid muscle
7 Body of axis (second cervical vertebra)	**14** External acoustic canal	**22** Inferior cerebellar vermis	**31** Lateral pterygoid plate
	15 External carotid artery	**23** Inferior nasal concha	**32** Left cerebellar hemisphere
		24 Inferior oblique muscle	

33 Levator labii superioris alaeque nasi muscle	**47** Nasopharynx	**59** Pharyngobasilar fascia	**73** Splenius capitis muscle
34 Levator veli palatini muscle	**48** Occipital condyle	**60** Pinna of ear	**74** Sternocleidomastoid muscle
35 Lingual septum	**49** Odontoid process (dens)	**61** Posterior arch of atlas	**75** Stylopharyngeus muscle
36 Longus capitis muscle	**50** Oropharynx	**62** Posterior belly of digastric muscle	**76** Subcutaneous fat
37 Marrow of clivus	**51** Palatine tonsils	**63** Posterior pharyngeal wall	**77** Submandibular gland
38 Masseter muscle	**52** Palatopharyngeus muscle	**64** Pterygomaxillary fissure	**78** Temporalis muscle
39 Mastoid process	**53** Parapharyngeal space	**65** Ramus of mandible	**79** Tensor veli palatini muscle
40 Maxillary sinus (antrum)	**54** Parotid duct	**66** Rectus capitis anterior muscle	**80** Trapezius muscle
41 Maxillary tuberosity	**55** Parotid gland	**67** Rectus capitis muscle	**81** Uvula
42 Medial pterygoid muscle	**56** Petrous portion of temporal bone	**68** Retromandibular vein	**82** Vertebral artery
43 Medial pterygoid plate	**57** Pharyngeal cartilaginous end of auditory tube (torus tubarius)	**69** Root of upper molar tooth	**83** Vomer
44 Medulla oblongata		**70** Semispinalis capitis muscle	**84** Zygomatic arch
45 Mylohyoid muscle		**71** Soft palate	**85** Zygomaticus muscle
46 Nasal septal cartilage	**58** Pharyngeal constrictor muscle	**72** Spinal cord	

(a)–(d) Nasopharynx and oropharynx, sagittal MR images.

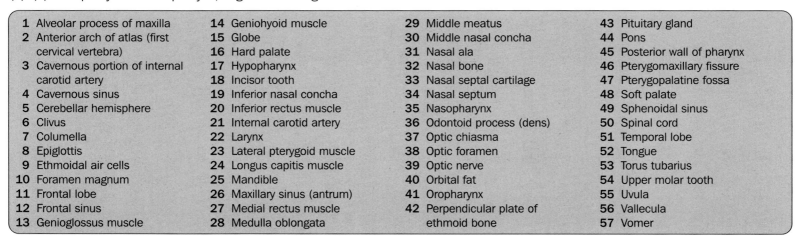

1 Alveolar process of maxilla	14 Geniohyoid muscle	29 Middle meatus	43 Pituitary gland
2 Anterior arch of atlas (first cervical vertebra)	15 Globe	30 Middle nasal concha	44 Pons
3 Cavernous portion of internal carotid artery	16 Hard palate	31 Nasal ala	45 Posterior wall of pharynx
	17 Hypopharynx	32 Nasal bone	46 Pterygomaxillary fissure
	18 Incisor tooth	33 Nasal septal cartilage	47 Pterygopalatine fossa
4 Cavernous sinus	19 Inferior nasal concha	34 Nasal septum	48 Soft palate
5 Cerebellar hemisphere	20 Inferior rectus muscle	35 Nasopharynx	49 Sphenoidal sinus
6 Clivus	21 Internal carotid artery	36 Odontoid process (dens)	50 Spinal cord
7 Columella	22 Larynx	37 Optic chiasma	51 Temporal lobe
8 Epiglottis	23 Lateral pterygoid muscle	38 Optic foramen	52 Tongue
9 Ethmoidal air cells	24 Longus capitis muscle	39 Optic nerve	53 Torus tubarius
10 Foramen magnum	25 Mandible	40 Orbital fat	54 Upper molar tooth
11 Frontal lobe	26 Maxillary sinus (antrum)	41 Oropharynx	55 Uvula
12 Frontal sinus	27 Medial rectus muscle	42 Perpendicular plate of ethmoid bone	56 Vallecula
13 Genioglossus muscle	28 Medulla oblongata		57 Vomer

(a)–(d) Nasopharynx and oropharynx, coronal MR images.

1 Anterior belly of digastric muscle	**12** Head of mandible	**23** Mylohyoid muscle	**34** Retromandibular vein
2 Anterior facial vein	**13** Internal carotid artery	**24** Nasopharynx	**35** Soft palate
3 Clivus	**14** Lateral pterygoid muscle	**25** Opening of auditory (Eustachian) tube	**36** Sphenoidal sinus
4 Coronoid process of mandible	**15** Lateral pterygoid plate	**26** Optic chiasma	**37** Stylopharyngeus muscle
5 Deep lobe of parotid gland	**16** Levator veli palatini muscle and tensor veli palatini muscle	**27** Palatal constrictor muscles	**38** Submandibular gland
6 Epiglottis	**17** Lingual artery	**28** Palatine artery	**39** Superficial lobe of parotid gland
7 Facial artery	**18** Longus capitis muscle	**29** Pituitary stalk	**40** Temporomandibular joint
8 Fat in parapharyngeal space	**19** Masseter muscle	**30** Platysma muscle	**41** Tongue
9 Genioglossus muscle	**20** Maxillary artery	**31** Pterygoid (vidian) canal	**42** Torus tubarius
10 Geniohyoid muscle	**21** Medial pterygoid muscle	**32** Pterygoid process of sphenoid	**43** Uvula
11 Hard palate	**22** Median raphe of tongue	**33** Ramus of mandible	**44** Vallecula

(a) Soft tissues of the neck, lateral projection.

1	Air in nasopharynx	9	Retropharyngeal soft tissues
2	Arytenoid cartilage	10	Sinus of larynx
3	Body of hyoid bone	11	Soft palate
4	Cricoid cartilage	12	Superior horn of thyroid cartilage
5	Cuneiform cartilage	13	Trachea
6	Epiglottis	14	Vallecula
7	Greater horn of hyoid bone	15	Vestibular fold
8	Posterior aspect of tongue	16	Vocal fold

(b) The kiss, sagittal MR image.

1 Deltoid insertion of levator muscle
2 Mandible
3 Nose
4 Pars marginalis of orbicularis oris muscle
5 Pars peripheralis of orbicularis oris muscle
6 Tongue

(c) Soft tissues of the neck, sagittal MR image.

1 Anterior arch of atlas (first cervical vertebra)
2 Anterior longitudinal ligament
3 Base of tongue
4 Body of seventh cervical vertebra
5 Cerebellar tonsil
6 Cerebrospinal fluid
7 Clivus
8 Epiglottis
9 Hypopharynx
10 Intervertebral disc (between fifth and sixth cervical vertebrae)
11 Medulla oblongata
12 Nasopharynx
13 Odontoid process (dens)
14 Oropharynx
15 Posterior arch of atlas (first cervical vertebra)
16 Posterior longitudinal ligament
17 Soft palate
18 Spinal cord
19 Spinous process of axis (second cervical vertebra)
20 Trachea

(d) and (e) Thyroid ultrasound, axial projection.

1 Deep cervical fascia
2 Internal jugular vein
3 Sternocleidomastoid muscle
4 Strap muscles of the neck
5 Thyroid gland
6 Thyroid isthmus

Tomography of the larynx, **(a)** at rest, **(b)** while phonating.

• Note how the vocal folds (7) move closer together during phonation.

1 Piriform fossa
2 Sinus of larynx
3 Thyroid cartilage
4 Trachea
5 Vestibular fold
6 Vestibule
7 Vocal fold

(c) and **(d)** Soft tissues of the neck, coronal MR images.

1	Apex of lung	14	Left parotid gland
2	Body of first thoracic vertebra	15	Left submandibular gland
3	Body of mandible	16	Left vertebral artery
4	Brachial plexus	17	Masseter muscle
5	Brachiocephalic trunk	18	Medial pterygoid muscle
6	Deep cervical fascia	19	Odontoid process (dens)
7	Inferior constrictor muscle	20	Platysma muscle
8	Inferior end plate of second thoracic vertebra	21	Right common carotid artery
9	Internal jugular vein	22	Scalenus medius muscle
10	Intervertebral disc (between sixth and seventh cervical vertebrae)	23	Sternocleidomastoid muscle
11	Lateral mass of atlas (first cervical vertebra)	24	Tongue
12	Lateral pterygoid muscle	25	Trachea
13	Left lobe of thyroid gland	26	Transverse process of first thoracic vertebra

(a)–(h) Larynx and hypopharynx, axial MR images.

1 Anterior belly of digastric muscle	**9** Body of mandible	**17** External jugular vein
2 Anterior commissure	**10** Cervical oesophagus	**18** Genioglossus muscle
3 Anterior jugular vein	**11** Common carotid artery	**19** Geniohyoid muscle
4 Anterior margin of cricoid cartilage	**12** Cricothyroid joint	**20** Glottic space
5 Aryepiglottic fold	**13** Deep cervical fascia	**21** Hyoglossus muscle
6 Arytenoid cartilage	**14** Epiglottic valleculae	**22** Hyoid bone
7 Base of tongue and epiglottis	**15** Epiglottis	**23** Hypopharynx
8 Body of fifth cervical vertebra	**16** External carotid artery	**24** Inferior horn of thyroid cartilage

25 Inferior oblique muscle	**41** Oropharynx	**56** Sternocleidomastoid muscle
26 Infrahyoid muscle	**42** Pharyngeal constrictor	**57** Subcutaneous fat
27 Internal carotid artery	**43** Platysma muscle	**58** Subglottic space
28 Internal jugular vein	**44** Posterior belly of digastric muscle	**59** Sublingual gland
29 Intrinsic tongue muscle	**45** Pre-epiglottic space	**60** Submandibular gland
30 Lamina of cricoid cartilage	**46** Prevertebral space	**61** Suprahyoid muscles
31 Laryngeal inlet	**47** Pyriform sinus	**62** Thyroid cartilage
32 Laryngeal vestibule	**48** Right lobe of thyroid	**63** Thyroid notch
33 Left lobe of thyroid	**49** Scalenus anterior muscle	**64** Trachea
34 Levator scapulae muscle	**50** Scalenus medius and posterior	**65** Tracheal ring
35 Lingual septum	muscles	**66** Trapezius muscle
36 Lingual tonsils	**51** Semispinalis capitis muscle	**67** Vertebral artery
37 Longus capitis muscle	**52** Semispinalis cervicis muscle	**68** Vertebral body
38 Longus colli muscle	**53** Semispinalis muscle	**69** Vestibular fold (false cord)
39 Multifidus muscle	**54** Spinal cord	**70** Vocal cord
40 Mylohyoid muscle	**55** Splenius capitis muscle	

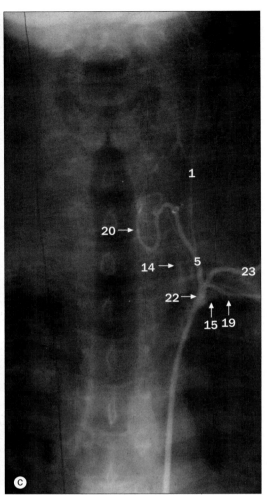

Digitally subtracted arteriograms of the external carotid artery, (a) anteroposterior projection, (b) lateral projection. (c) Thyroid arteriogram.

1 Ascending cervical artery	**11** Occipital artery	**19** Suprascapular artery
2 Ascending pharyngeal artery	**12** Posterior auricular artery	**20** Thyroid branches of
3 Endotracheal tube	**13** Posterior superior alveolar	inferior thyroid artery
4 Facial artery	artery	**21** Tip of catheter in external
5 Inferior thyroid artery	**14** Reflux of contrast into	carotid artery
6 Infra-orbital artery	vertebral artery	**22** Tip of catheter in
7 Labial branch of facial artery	**15** Subclavian artery	thyrocervical trunk
8 Lingual artery	**16** Submental artery	**23** Transverse cervical artery
9 Maxillary artery	**17** Superficial temporal artery	
10 Middle meningeal artery	**18** Superior thyroid artery	

(d) Neck venogram, (e) MR angiogram of neck vessels.

1	Common carotid artery
2	External carotid artery
3	Inferior thyroid vein
4	Internal carotid artery
5	Internal jugular vein
6	Lingual vein
7	Superior thyroid vein
8	Tip of catheter in middle thyroid vein
9	Vertebral artery

(a) Parotid sialogram. ▼

1 Catheter	**4** Mandible
2 Coronoid process of mandible	**5** Mastoid process
	6 Parotid (Stensen's) duct
3 Hyoid bone	**7** Secondary ductules

(c) Parotid sialogram, submentovertical projection. ▲

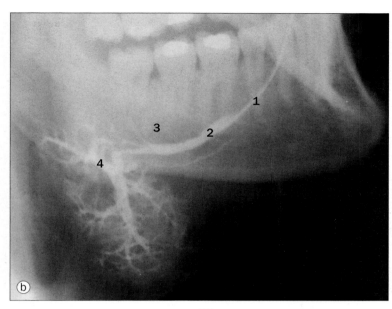

(b) Submandibular sialogram. ▼

1 Catheter
2 Main submandibular (Wharton's) duct
3 Mandible
4 Secondary ductules

(d) Orthopantomogram. ▼

1 Alveolar process of maxilla	**12** Inferior alveolar canal
2 Anterior nasal spine	**13** Lamina propria
3 Canine	**14** Lateral incisor
4 Central incisor	**15** Maxillary sinus (antrum)
5 Condyle of mandible	**16** Mental foramen
6 Coronoid process of mandible	**17** Pulp chamber
7 External acoustic meatus	**18** Second molar
8 First molar	**19** Second premolar
9 First premolar	**20** Temporomandibular joint
10 Hard palate	**21** Third molar
11 Hyoid bone	

Orbits, axial CT images are demonstrated at the following levels: **(a)** inferior orbit and globe; **(b)** mid orbit below the optic nerve; **(c)** mid orbit at the level of the optic nerve; **(d)** superior orbit.

1 Angular vein	**11** Frontal bone	**21** Lacrimal sac
2 Anterior chamber	**12** Frontal sinus	**22** Lacrimal vein
3 Anterior clinoid process	**13** Greater wing of sphenoid	**23** Lamina papyracea
4 Brainstem	**14** Inferior nasal concha (turbinate)	**24** Lateral rectus muscle
5 Cavernous sinus	**15** Inferior oblique muscle	**25** Lens
6 Crista galli	**16** Inferior orbital fissure	**26** Lesser wing of sphenoid
7 Dorsum sellae	**17** Inferior rectus muscle	**27** Levator palpebrae superioris muscle
8 Ethmoidal sinuses	**18** Infra-orbital canal	**28** Long posterior ciliary artery
9 Ethmoidal sinuses (posterior)	**19** Infra-orbital margin	**29** Maxillary sinus (antrum)
10 Eyelid	**20** Lacrimal gland	**30** Medial ophthalmic vein

Orbits, coronal CT images are demonstrated at the following levels: **(e)** globe, **(f)** mid orbit, **(g)** posterior orbit, **(h)** superior and inferior orbital fissures.

31 Medial rectus muscle	**41** Petrous ridge	**51** Superior ophthalmic vein
32 Middle nasal concha (turbinate)	**42** Pituitary gland	**52** Superior orbital fissure
33 Nasal bone	**43** Planum sphenoidale	**53** Superior rectus muscle
34 Nasal cavity	**44** Pterygopalatine fossa	**54** Supra-orbital margin
35 Nasal septum	**45** Retrobulbar fat	**55** Temporal lobe
36 Nasolacrimal duct	**46** Sclera	**56** Temporalis muscle
37 Ophthalmic artery	**47** Sphenoidal sinus	**57** Trochlea of superior oblique muscle
38 Optic canal	**48** Superior nasal concha (turbinate)	**58** Vitreous
39 Optic nerve	**49** Superior oblique muscle	**59** Zygomatic bone
40 Orbicularis muscle	**50** Superior oblique tendon	**60** Zygomatic process of frontal bone

Digitally subtracted arterial phase of carotid arteriograms,
(a) anteroposterior projection, (b) lateral projection, (c) oblique
projection.

(a) Digitally subtracted venous phase of carotid arteriogram, anteroposterior projection.

1 Basal vein of Rosenthal
2 Inferior sagittal sinus
3 Internal cerebral vein
4 Internal jugular vein
5 Jugular bulb
6 Right transverse sinus
7 Superficial cortical veins
8 Superior sagittal sinus
9 Thalamostriate vein

(b) Digitally subtracted venous phase of carotid arteriogram, lateral projection.

 1 Anterior caudate vein
 2 Basal vein of Rosenthal
 3 Cavernous sinus
 4 Confluence of venous sinuses (torcular Herophili)
 5 Great cerebral vein of Galen
 6 Inferior sagittal sinus
 7 Internal cerebral vein
 8 Internal jugular vein
 9 Sigmoid sinus
10 Sphenoparietal sinus
11 Straight sinus
12 Superficial cerebral veins
13 Superior sagittal sinus
14 Thalamostriate vein
15 Transverse sinus
16 Vein of Labbé
17 Vein of Trolard
18 Venous angle

(a) Digitally subtracted arterial phase of vertebral arteriogram, anteroposterior projection.

1 Anterior inferior cerebellar artery
2 Anterior spinal artery
3 Basilar artery
4 Calcarine artery
5 Hemispheric branch of superior cerebellar artery
6 Inferior temporal artery
7 Medullary segment of posterior inferior cerebellar artery
8 Parieto-occipital artery
9 Posterior cerebral artery in ambient cistern
10 Posterior cerebral artery in interpeduncular cistern
11 Posterior inferior cerebellar artery
12 Quadrigeminal portion of posterior cerebral artery
13 Site of junction with posterior communicating artery
14 Superior cerebellar arteries behind brainstem
15 Superior cerebellar artery
16 Thalamoperforating branches of superior cerebellar artery
17 Vermian branch of superior cerebellar artery
18 Vertebral artery exiting transverse foramen of atlas (first cervical vertebra)

(b) Digitally subtracted arterial phase of vertebral arteriogram, lateral projection.

1 Anterior inferior cerebellar artery
2 Anterior medullary segment of posterior inferior cerebellar artery
3 Basilar artery
4 Calcarine artery
5 Hemispheric branches of posterior inferior cerebellar artery
6 Inferior vermian segment of posterior inferior cerebellar artery
7 Lateral medullary segment of posterior inferior cerebellar artery
8 Meningeal branch of vertebral artery
9 Origin of posterior inferior cerebellar artery
10 Parieto-occipital artery
11 Posterior cerebral artery
12 Posterior choroidal branches of posterior cerebral artery
13 Posterior medullary segment of posterior inferior cerebellar artery
14 Posterior temporal artery
15 Retrotonsillar segment of posterior inferior cerebellar artery
16 Splenial branches of posterior cerebral artery
17 Superior cerebellar artery
18 Supratonsillar segment of posterior inferior cerebellar artery
19 Thalamoperforate branches of posterior cerebral artery
20 Vertebral artery
21 Vertebral artery exiting transverse foramen of atlas (first cervical vertebra)

(a) Digitally subtracted venous phase of vertebral arteriogram, anteroposterior projection.

1	Anterior pontomesencephalic vein
2	Inferior hemispheric vein
3	Inferior vermian vein
4	Internal jugular vein
5	Jugular bulb
6	Left transverse sinus
7	Petrosal vein
8	Posterior mesencephalic vein
9	Right transverse sinus
10	Straight sinus
11	Superior hemispheric vein
12	Superior petrosal sinus

(b) Digitally subtracted venous phase of vertebral arteriogram, lateral projection.

1	Anterior pontomesencephalic vein
2	Confluence of venous sinuses (torcular Herophili)
3	Great cerebral vein of Galen
4	Inferior hemispheric vein
5	Inferior vermian vein
6	Internal jugular vein
7	Jugular bulb
8	Lateral mesencephalic vein
9	Posterior mesencephalic vein
10	Precentral cerebellar vein
11	Sigmoid sinus
12	Straight sinus
13	Superior choroidal vein
14	Superior hemispheric vein
15	Superior vermian vein
16	Tonsillar vein
17	Transverse sinus
18	Vein of the great horizontal fissure

Circle of Willis, arteries of the brain with MRA, **(a)** axial and **(b)** lateral projection.

1 Anterior cerebral artery	**10** Ophthalmic artery
2 Anterior communicating artery	**11** Petrous portion of internal carotid artery
3 Basilar artery	**12** Posterior cerebral artery
4 Branches (in insula) of middle cerebral artery	**13** Posterior cerebral artery in ambient cistern
5 Cavernous portion of internal carotid artery	**14** Posterior cerebral artery in interpeduncular cistern
6 Cervical portion of internal carotid artery	**15** Posterior communicating artery
7 Genu of middle cerebral artery	**16** Posterior inferior cerebellar artery
8 Intracranial (supraclinoid) internal carotid artery	**17** Quadrigeminal portion of posterior cerebral artery
9 Middle cerebral artery	**18** Superior cerebellar artery

Circle of Willis, MRA veins of the brain, **(a)** lateral projection,
(b) axial projection.

1 Basal vein of Rosenthal	**9** Internal cerebral vein
2 Basilar artery	**10** Left transverse sinus
3 Cavernous sinus	**11** Right transverse sinus
4 Confluence of venous sinuses (torcular Herophili)	**12** Sphenoparietal sinus
5 Great cerebral vein of Galen	**13** Straight sinus
6 Inferior petrosal sinus	**14** Superficial cerebral veins
7 Inferior sagittal sinus	**15** Superior petrosal sinus
8 Internal carotid artery	**16** Superior sagittal sinus

(a)–(l) Brain, axial MR images.

1 Ambient cistern	**11** Centrum semi ovale	Herophili)
2 Anterior cerebral artery	**12** Cerebellar folia	**22** Corona radiata
3 Anterior limb of internal capsule	**13** Cerebellar tonsil	**23** Cortical vein
4 Aqueduct of Sylvius	**14** Cerebellopontine cistern	**24** Dentate nucleus
5 Basilar artery	**15** Cerebral peduncle	**25** Diploe
6 Body of lateral ventricle	**16** Choroid plexus in trigone of lateral ventricle	**26** Dorsum sellae
7 Branch of middle cerebral artery in lateral	**17** Choroid vessels	**27** Ethmoidal air cells
sulcus (Sylvian fissure)	**18** Cingulate gyrus	**28** External acoustic meatus
8 Callosomarginal artery	**19** Claustrum	**29** External capsule
9 Caudate nucleus	**20** Cochlea	**30** Facial nerve in internal acoustic canal
10 Central sulcus of Rolando	**21** Confluence of venous sinuses (torcular	

31 Falx cerebri	41 Globus pallidus	51 Insular gyri
32 Forceps major	42 Grey matter	52 Internal acoustic meatus
33 Forceps minor	43 Head of caudate nucleus	53 Internal carotid artery
34 Fornix	44 Inferior cerebellar peduncle	54 Internal cerebral vein
35 Fourth ventricle	45 Inferior cerebellar vermis	55 Interpeduncular cistern
36 Frontal horn of lateral ventricle	46 Inferior colliculus	56 Interventricular foramen of Monro
37 Frontal lobe	47 Inferior sagittal sinus	57 Lateral rectus muscle
38 Frontal sinus	48 Inferior(temporal) horn of lateral ventricle	58 Lateral sulcus (Sylvian fissure)
39 Genu of corpus callosum	49 Inner table, dura and cerebrospinal fluid	59 Left cerebellar hemisphere
40 Globe	50 Insula	60 Lens

(i)–(p) Brain, axial MR images.

61 Mammillary bodies in suprasellar cistern	73 Optic nerve	85 Posterior limb of internal capsule
62 Mastoid air cells	74 Optic radiations	86 Posterior(occipital) horn of lateral ventricle
63 Maxillary sinus (antrum)	75 Optic tract	87 Precentral gyrus
64 Medial rectus muscle	76 Outer table	88 Prepontine cistern
65 Medulla oblongata	77 Parahippocampal gyrus	89 Putamen
66 Mesencephalon (midbrain)	78 Petrous temporal bone	90 Pyramid of medulla oblongata
67 Middle cerebellar peduncle	79 Pinna of ear	91 Quadrigeminal cistern
68 Middle cerebral artery	80 Pituitary gland	92 Red nucleus
69 Nasal septum	81 Pons	93 Retro-orbital fat
70 Nodule of cerebellum	82 Postcentral gyrus	94 Septum pellucidum
71 Occipital lobe	83 Posterior cerebral artery	95 Sigmoid sinus
72 Optic chiasma in suprasellar cistern	84 Posterior cerebral artery in ambient cistern	

96 Sphenoidal sinus
97 Splenium of corpus callosum
98 Straight sinus
99 Substantia nigra
100 Superficial temporal artery
101 Superior cerebellar peduncle
102 Superior cerebellar vermis
103 Superior colliculus
104 Superior frontal gyrus
105 Superior ophthalmic vein
106 Superior sagittal sinus

107 Superior vermis
108 Temporal lobe
109 Thalamus
110 Third ventricle
111 Trigone of lateral ventricle
112 Vagus nerve
113 Vertebral artery
114 Vestibular part of inner ear
115 Vestibulocochlear nerve in internal acoustic canal
116 White matter

(a)–(d) Brain, sagittal MR images.

1 Alveolar ridge	**15** Cisterna magna	**29** Internal cerebral vein	**43** Pituitary gland
2 Anterior arch of atlas (first	(cerebellomedullary cistern)	**30** Interventricular foramen of	**44** Pons
cervical vertebra)	**16** Corona radiata	Monro	**45** Posterior arch of atlas
3 Anterior cerebral artery	**17** Cortical vein	**31** Lateral ventricle	**46** Prepontine cistern
4 Basilar artery	**18** Foramen magnum	**32** Lentiform nucleus	**47** Sphenoidal sinus
5 Body of corpus callosum	**19** Fourth ventricle	**33** Mandible	**48** Splenium of corpus callosum
6 Body of lateral ventricle	**20** Frontal sinus	**34** Maxillary sinus (antrum)	**49** Superior cerebellar peduncle
7 Central sulcus of Rolando	**21** Genu of corpus callosum	**35** Medulla oblongata	**50** Superior colliculus
8 Cerebellar folia	**22** Globe	**36** Middle cerebellar peduncle	**51** Sylvian fissure
9 Cerebellar hemisphere	**23** Great cerebral vein of Galen	**37** Middle cerebral artery	**52** Tegmentum of pons
10 Cerebellum	**24** Head of caudate nucleus	**38** Nasopharynx	**53** Temporal lobe of brain
11 Cerebral peduncle	**25** Inferior cerebellar peduncle	**39** Odontoid process (dens)	**54** Tentorium cerebelli
12 Cervical spinal cord	**26** Inferior colliculus	**40** Optic chiasma in suprasellar	**55** Third ventricle
13 Cingulate gyrus	**27** Inferior rectus muscle	cistern	**56** Vertebral artery
14 Cingulate sulcus	**28** Internal carotid artery in	**41** Optic nerve	
	cavernous sinus	**42** Orbital cortex of frontal lobe	

Brain, sagittal MR midline image.

1 Anterior arch of atlas (first cervical vertebra)	15 Fat in marrow of clivus	31 Parieto-occipital fissure
2 Anterior cerebral artery	16 Foramen magnum	32 Pineal gland
3 Anterior commissure	17 Fornix	33 Pituitary gland
4 Aqueduct of Sylvius	18 Fourth ventricle	34 Pons
5 Basilar artery	19 Frontal sinus	35 Posterior arch of atlas
6 Body of corpus callosum	20 Genu of corpus callosum	36 Posterior commissure
7 Cerebellar folia	21 Great cerebral vein of Galen	37 Prepontine cistern
8 Cerebellar tonsil	22 Internal cerebral vein	38 Quadrigeminal cistern
9 Cerebellum	23 Interventricular foramen of Monro	39 Quadrigeminal plate of midbrain
10 Cerebral peduncles of midbrain	24 Lamina terminalis	40 Sphenoidal sinus
11 Cervical spinal cord	25 Lateral ventricle	41 Splenium of corpus callosum
12 Cingulate gyrus	26 Mammillary body	42 Superior medullary velum
13 Cisterna magna (cerebellomedullary cistern)	27 Massa intermedia	43 Tegmentum of pons
	28 Medulla oblongata	44 Tentorium cerebelli
14 Diploic veins	29 Nasopharynx	45 Third ventricle
	30 Odontoid process (dens)	

(a)–(h) Brain, coronal MR images.

1 Ambient cistern	**11** Cisterna magna (cerebellomedullary cistern)	**21** Interhemispheric cistern
2 Aqueduct of Sylvius	**12** Claustrum and external capsule	**22** Internal capsule
3 Atlas (first cervical vertebra)	**13** External capsule	**23** Interpeduncular cistern
4 Body of caudate nucleus	**14** Fornix	**24** Intracavernous internal carotid artery
5 Body of corpus callosum	**15** Fourth ventricle	**25** Lateral ventricle
6 Body of lateral ventricle	**16** Head of caudate nucleus	**26** Lentiform nucleus
7 Cavum septum pellucidum	**17** Hippocampus	**27** Mandible
8 Cerebellar hemisphere	**18** Inferior colliculus	**28** Marrow of basisphenoid (clivus)
9 Cerebral peduncle	**19** Inferior(temporal) horn of lateral ventricle	**29** Medulla oblongata
10 Choroid plexus	**20** Insula	**30** Middle cerebellar peduncle

31 Nodule of cerebellum
32 Odontoid process (dens)
33 Optic chiasma in suprasellar cistern
34 Optic nerve
35 Optic tract
36 Pineal gland
37 Pituitary gland
38 Pituitary stalk in suprasellar cistern
39 Pons
40 Prepontine cistern

41 Quadrigeminal cistern
42 Sigmoid sinus
43 Sphenoidal sinus
44 Splenium of corpus callosum
45 Superior colliculus
46 Superior sagittal sinus
47 Superior vermis
48 Supraclinoid internal carotid artery
49 Suprapineal recess of the third ventricle
50 Suprasellar cistern

51 Sylvian fissure
52 Temporal lobe
53 Tentorium cerebelli
54 Thalamus
55 Third ventricle
56 Trigeminal (gasserian) ganglion in recess (Meckel's cave)
57 Trigeminal nerve
58 Trigone of lateral ventricle

(a)–(d) Neonatal brain, coronal ultrasound images.

 1 Body of caudate nucleus
 2 Brainstem
 3 Cavum septum pellucidum
 4 Cerebellum
 5 Choroid plexus
 6 Corpus callosum
 7 Falx cerebri
 8 Head of caudate nucleus
 9 Lateral ventricle
10 Parietal lobe of brain
11 Sylvian fissure
12 Temporal lobe
13 Thalamus
14 Third ventricle

(e)–(h) Neonatal brain, sagittal ultrasound images.

1 Body of caudate nucleus	**11** Greater wing of sphenoid
2 Body of corpus callosum	**12** Head of caudate nucleus
3 Brainstem	**13** Lateral ventricle
4 Cavum septum pellucidum	**14** Occipital lobe
5 Cerebellum	**15** Parietal lobe of brain
6 Choroid plexus	**16** Splenium of corpus callosum
7 Clivus	**17** Temporal lobe
8 Fourth ventricle	**18** Thalamus
9 Frontal lobe	**19** Third ventricle
10 Genu of corpus callosum	

(a)–(d) Pituitary fossa (sella turcica), coronal CT images.
These images show 2 mm coronal slices through the sella turcica (pituitary fossa) from anterior (a) to posterior (d) during the intravenous infusion of non-ionic water-soluble contrast medium.

1 Anterior cerebral artery	**13** Lateral pterygoid plate	**24** Pituitary gland
2 Anterior clinoid process	**14** Lateral sulcus (Sylvian fissure) with	**25** Pituitary stalk
3 Body of fornix	branches of middle cerebral artery	**26** Pterygoid (vidian) canal
4 Cavernous carotid artery	**15** Lateral ventricle	**27** Sphenoidal sinus
5 Cavernous sinus	**16** Medial pterygoid muscle	**28** Supraclinoid internal carotid artery
6 Choroid plexus	**17** Medial pterygoid plate	**29** Suprasellar cistern
7 Dorsum sellae	**18** Middle cerebral artery	**30** Temporal lobe of brain
8 Floor of middle cranial fossa	**19** Nasopharynx	**31** Third ventricle
9 Floor of pituitary fossa (sella turcica)	**20** Oculomotor nerve	**32** Torus tubarius
10 Foramen lacerum	**21** Optic chiasma	**33** Trigeminal (gasserian) ganglion in recess
11 Foramen ovale	**22** Orifice of auditory (Eustachian) tube	(Meckel's cave)
12 Lateral pterygoid muscle	**23** Pharyngeal recess (fossa of Rosenmuller)	**34** Trigeminal nerve

Pituitary fossa (sella turcica), coronal MR images, (a) at the level of the anterior clinoid, (b) mid fossa, (c) at the level of the pituitary stalk, (d) at the level of the dorsum sellae.

1 Anterior cerebral artery	**9** Internal carotid artery in cavernous sinus	**18** Pituitary stalk
2 Anterior horn of lateral ventricle	**10** Lateral pterygoid muscle	**19** Posterior clinoid process
3 Bifurcation of internal carotid artery	**11** Lateral sulcus (Sylvian fissure)	**20** Septum pellucidum
4 Branch of middle cerebral artery in lateral sulcus (Sylvian fissure)	**12** Medial pterygoid muscle	**21** Sphenoidal sinus
5 Cingulate gyrus	**13** Nasopharynx	**22** Supraclinoid carotid artery
6 Corpus callosum	**14** Optic chiasma	**23** Suprasellar cistern
7 Insula	**15** Optic tract	**24** Temporal lobe of brain
8 Interhemispheric fissure	**16** Parietal lobe of brain	**25** Temporalis muscle
	17 Pituitary gland	**26** Third ventricle

(a)–(d) Pituitary fossa, sagittal MR images.

1 Anterior pituitary gland	**9** Medulla oblongata	**17** Quadrigeminal cistern
2 Aqueduct of Sylvius	**10** Optic chiasma in suprasellar cistern	**18** Quadrigeminal plate of midbrain
3 Body of corpus callosum	**11** Optic tract	**19** Sphenoidal sinus
4 Fat in marrow of clivus	**12** Pituitary stalk	**20** Splenium of corpus callosum
5 Fourth ventricle	**13** Pons	**21** Suprasellar cistern
6 Genu of corpus callosum	**14** Posterior clinoid process	**22** Thalamus
7 Lateral ventricle	**15** Posterior pituitary gland	
8 Mammillary body	**16** Prepontine cistern	

(a)–(d) Pituitary fossa, sagittal MR images, post gadolinium.

1 Anterior pituitary gland
2 Aqueduct of Sylvius
3 Cavernous portion of internal carotid artery
4 Cavernous sinus
5 Cisterna magna (cerebellomedullary cistern)
6 Fourth ventricle
7 Great cerebral vein of Galen
8 Interpeduncular cistern
9 Mammillary body
10 Optic chiasma
11 Optic tract
12 Pituitary stalk
13 Posterior clinoid process
14 Posterior pituitary gland
15 Prepontine cistern
16 Suprasellar cistern
17 Thalamus

2 Vertebral column and spinal cord

(a) Cervical spine, anteroposterior projection.

(b) Dried cervical vertebra, anteroposterior projection.

1 Body of vertebra
2 Inferior articular process (facet)
3 Intertubercular lamella of transverse process
4 Posterior tubercle of transverse process
5 Posterolateral lip (uncus)
6 Region of vocal cords
7 Spinous process
8 Superior articular process (facet)
9 Trachea

(c) Cervical spine, lateral projection;
(d) dried atlas (first cervical vertebra), lateral projection; **(e)** dried axis (second cervical vertebra), lateral projection; **(f)** dried fourth cervical vertebra, lateral projection.

1 Anterior arch of atlas (first cervical vertebra)
2 Anterior tubercle of transverse process of fourth cervical vertebra
3 Body of axis (second cervical vertebra)
4 Inferior articular process (facet) of fourth cervical vertebra
5 Odontoid process (dens) of axis (second cervical vertebra)
6 Posterior arch of atlas (first cervical vertebra)
7 Posterior tubercle of atlas (first cervical vertebra)
8 Posterior tubercle of transverse process of fourth cervical vertebra
9 Spinous process of atlas (first cervical vertebra)
10 Spinous process of axis (second cervical vertebra)
11 Spinous process of fourth cervical vertebra
12 Superior articular process (facet) of fourth cervical vertebra

(a) Atlas (first cervical vertebra) and axis (second cervical vertebra), 'open mouth' anteroposterior projection.
(b) Dried atlas (first cervical vertebra), anteroposterior projection.
(c) Dried axis (second cervical vertebra), anteroposterior projection.
(d) Cervical spine of a 3-year-old child, lateral projection.
• The apparent widening of the atlanto-axial joint (2) is a normal feature at this age.
(e) Cervical spine, oblique projection.

1   Anterior arch of atlas (first cervical vertebra)
2   Atlanto-axial joint of axis (second cervical vertebra)
3   Bifid spinous process of axis (second cervical vertebra)
4   Body of axis (second cervical vertebra)
5   Body of fifth cervical vertebra
6   Hyoid bone
7   Inferior articular process (facet) of atlas (first cervical vertebra)
8   Intervertebral foramen
9   Lamina of fifth cervical vertebra
10 Lateral mass of atlas (first cervical vertebra)

11 Left first rib
12 Mandible
13 Occipital bone
14 Odontoid process (dens) of axis (second cervical vertebra)
15 Posterior tubercle of transverse process of fifth cervical vertebra
16 Posterolateral lip (uncus) of fifth cervical vertebra
17 Right first rib
18 Spinous process of fifth cervical vertebra
19 Superior articular process (facet) of atlas (first cervical vertebra)
20 Superior articular process (facet) of axis (second cervical vertebra)
21 Trachea
22 Transverse process of atlas (first cervical vertebra)
23 Transverse process of axis (second cervical vertebra)
24 Transverse process of fifth cervical vertebra

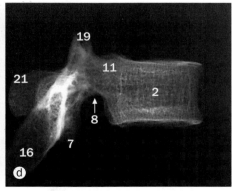

1 Body of sixth thoracic vertebra
2 Body of vertebra
3 Clavicle
4 First rib
5 First thoracic vertebra
6 Inferior annular epiphysial discs for vertebral body
7 Inferior articular process (facet)
8 Inferior vertebral notch
9 Left main bronchus
10 Neonatal cleft
11 Pedicle
12 Pedicle of sixth thoracic vertebra
13 Ribs
14 Right main bronchus
15 Site of intervertebral disc
16 Spinous process
17 Spinous process of sixth thoracic vertebra
18 Superior annular epiphysial discs for vertebral body
19 Superior articular process (facet)
20 Trachea
21 Transverse process
22 Transverse process of sixth thoracic vertebra

(a) Thoracic spine, anteroposterior projection.

(b) Dried thoracic vertebra, anteroposterior projection.

(c) Thoracic spine, lateral projection.

(d) Dried sixth thoracic vertebra, lateral projection.

Thoracic spine, (e) of a 7-day-old neonate, (f) of a 12-year-old child, lateral projections.

(a) Lumbar spine, anteroposterior radiograph.

(b) Lumbar spine, lateral projection.

(c) Dried second lumbar vertebra, anteroposterior projection.

(d) Dried second lumbar vertebra, lateral projection.

(e) Lumbar spine, oblique projection.

1   Body of first lumbar vertebra
2   Body of second lumbar vertebra
3   Body of twelfth thoracic vertebra
4   Fifth lumbar vertebra
5   Inferior articular process (facet) of second lumbar vertebra
6   Inferior vertebral notch of second lumbar vertebra
7   Mammillary process of second lumbar vertebra
8   Pars interarticularis
9   Pedicle of second lumbar vertebra
10 Right twelfth rib
11 Sacral promontory
12 Spinous process of second lumbar vertebra
13 Superior articular process (facet) of second lumbar vertebra
14 Transverse process of second lumbar vertebra

(a)–(d) Cervical spine, axial CT images at the level of the atlas (first cervical vertebra).

1 Anterior arch of atlas (first cervical vertebra)	**11** Lateral mass of atlas (first cervical vertebra)	**18** Semispinalis capitis muscle
2 Anterior tubercle of atlas	**12** Odontoid process (dens) of axis (second cervical vertebra)	**19** Spinal cord
3 Articular pillar		**20** Spinous process of axis
4 Attachment of transverse ligament	**13** Pedicle	**21** Splenius capitis muscle
5 Body of axis (second cervical vertebra)	**14** Posterior arch of atlas (first cervical vertebra)	**22** Subarachnoid space
6 Epidural space		**23** Superior articular process (facet) of atlas (first cervical vertebra)
7 Groove for vertebral artery	**15** Posterior tubercle of atlas (first cervical vertebra)	
8 Inferior articular process (facet)		**24** Transverse foramen
9 Inferior oblique muscle	**16** Prevertebral soft tissue	**25** Transverse process
10 Lamina	**17** Rectus capitis muscle	**26** Vertebral artery in transverse foramen

(a)–(d) Cervical spine, axial CT images at the level of the fifth and sixth cervical vertebrae.

1	Airway at level of vocal cord	**9**	Intervertebral foramen	**18**	Spinous process
2	Anterior tubercle	**10**	Lamina	**19**	Spinous process of fourth cervical vertebra
3	Articular pillar	**11**	Multifidus muscle	**20**	Thyroid cartilage
4	Body of fifth cervical vertebra	**12**	Pedicle	**21**	Transverse foramen
5	Contrast medium in subarachnoid space	**13**	Posterior tubercle	**22**	Uncinate process
6	Cricoid cartilage	**14**	Pyriform sinus	**23**	Ventral ramus
7	Dorsal ramus	**15**	Semispinalis capitis muscle	**24**	Vocal cord
8	Intervertebral disc (between fifth and sixth cervical vertebra)	**16**	Semispinalis cervicis muscle		
		17	Spinal cord		

(a) and (b) Cervical spine, axial MR images.

1. Anterior longitudinal ligament and cortical bone
2. Body of vertebra
3. Cerebrospinal fluid in subarachnoid space
4. Common carotid artery
5. Dorsal ramus
6. Dorsal root ganglion
7. Epidural fat
8. Grey matter of cervical spinal cord
9. Inferior articular process (facet)
10. Internal jugular vein
11. Intervertebral foramen
12. Lamina
13. Levator scapulae muscle
14. Ligamentum flavum
15. Longus cervicis muscle
16. Multifidus muscle
17. Oesophagus
18. Posterior longitudinal ligament and cortical bone
19. Semispinalis capitis muscle
20. Spinous process
21. Splenius capitis muscle
22. Sternocleidomastoid muscle
23. Superior articular process (facet)
24. Thyroid gland
25. Trachea
26. Trapezius muscle
27. Ventral ramus
28. Vertebral artery in transverse foramen
29. White matter of cervical spinal cord
30. Zygapophysial (facet joint)

(a)–(d) Thoracic spine, axial CT images at the level of the sixth thoracic vertebra (with intrathecal contrast medium).

1	Anterior longitudinal ligament	**11**	Inferior articular process (facet) of sixth thoracic vertebra	**19**	Pedicle
2	Aorta			**20**	Right lung
3	Basivertebral veins	**12**	Intervertebral disc (between fifth and sixth thoracic vertebrae)	**21**	Spinal cord
4	Body of sixth thoracic vertebra			**22**	Spinous process
5	Contrast medium in subarachnoid space	**13**	Intervertebral foramen	**23**	Superior articular process (facet) of seventh thoracic vertebra
6	Costotransverse joint	**14**	Lamina		
7	Costovertebral joint	**15**	Left lung	**24**	Transverse process
8	Epidural space	**16**	Ligamentum flavum	**25**	Trapezius muscle
9	Erector spinae muscles	**17**	Neck of rib	**26**	Tubercle of rib
10	Head of rib	**18**	Oesophagus		

Spinal cord, (a) and (b) sagittal MR images.

1 Anterior arch of atlas (first cervical vertebra)	**15** Nucleus pulposus of intervertebral disc (between seventh cervical and first thoracic vertebrae)
2 Anterior longitudinal ligament and cortical bone	**16** Occipital bone
3 Basivertebral vein	**17** Odontoid process (dens)
4 Body of axis (second cervical vertebra)	**18** Oesophagus
5 Body of seventh cervical vertebra	**19** Posterior arch of atlas (first cervical vertebra)
6 Body of seventh thoracic vertebra	**20** Posterior longitudinal ligament
7 Brainstem	**21** Posterior longitudinal ligament and annulus fibrosus
8 Cerebellar tonsil	**22** Posterior longitudinal ligament and cortical bone
9 Cerebrospinal fluid in subarachnoid space	**23** Posterior margin of foramen magnum
10 Cervical expansion	**24** Spinal cord
11 Clivus	**25** Spinous process
12 Epidural fat	**26** Suboccipital fat
13 Ligamentum flavum	**27** Trachea
14 Nucleus pulposus of intervertebral disc (between seventh and eighth thoracic vertebrae)	

(a)–(d) Lumbar spine, axial CT images at the level of the fourth and fifth lumbar vertebrae (with intrathecal contrast medium).

Multiple thin (5 mm) sections are taken parallel to the disc space. Lumbar epidural fat provides contrast around the theca and exiting nerve roots, and the posterior aspect of the disc.

1 Annulus fibrosus of intervertebral disc	**10** Intervertebral foramen (between fourth and fifth lumbar vertebrae)	**19** Posterior longitudinal ligament
2 Anterior longitudinal ligament		**20** Psoas muscle
3 Basivertebral veins	**11** Lamina	**21** Right common iliac artery
4 Body of fourth lumbar vertebra	**12** Left common iliac artery	**22** Root of fourth lumbar nerve
5 Dorsal root ganglion of fourth lumbar nerve	**13** Ligamentum flavum	**23** Spinous process of fourth lumbar vertebra
6 Epidural fat	**14** Multifidus muscle	**24** Superior articular process (facet) of fifth
7 Erector spinae muscle	**15** Nerve roots of cauda equina	**25** Thecal sac
8 Inferior articular process (facet) of fourth lumbar vertebra	**16** Nucleus pulposus of intervertebral disc	**26** Transverse process
	17 Pars interarticularis	
9 Inferior vena cava	**18** Pedicle	

(a)–(d) Lumbar spine, axial CT images at the level of the lumbrosacral junction (with intrathecal contrast medium).

1 Body of fifth lumbar vertebra	**9** Internal vertebral veins	**18** Root of first sacral nerve
2 Body of sacrum	**10** Intervertebral disc (fifth lumbar/first sacral	**19** Sacral foramina
3 Bowel gas	vertebra)	**20** Sacro-iliac joint
4 Epidural fat	**11** Lamina	**21** Spinous process of fifth lumbar vertebra
5 Erector spinae muscle	**12** Lateral part (ala) of sacrum	**22** Spinous process of fourth lumbar vertebra
6 Ilium	**13** Ligamentum flavum	**23** Superior articular process (facet) of fifth
7 Inferior articular process (facet) of fifth	**14** Median sacral crest	lumbar vertebra)
lumbar vertebra	**15** Multifidus muscle	**24** Superior articular process (facet) of first
8 Inferior articular process (facet) of fourth	**16** Nerve roots of cauda equina	sacral vertebra
lumbar vertebra	**17** Root of fifth lumbar nerve	**25** Thecal sac

(a)–(e) Lumbar spine, axial MR images.

1	Annulus fibrosus and posterior longitudinal ligament	**14**	Lamina
2	Anterior longitudinal ligament and cortical bone	**15**	Ligamentum flavum
3	Aorta	**16**	Multifidus muscle
4	Cauda equina in lumbar thecal sac	**17**	Pedicle
5	Dorsal root ganglion	**18**	Posterior longitudinal ligament
6	Dura	**19**	Psoas muscle
7	Epidural fat in epidural space	**20**	Retroperitoneal fat
8	Epidural veins in epidural space	**21**	Spinal nerve root
9	Erector spinae muscles	**22**	Spinous process
10	Fat in intervertebral foramen	**23**	Superior articular process (facet)
11	Inferior articular process (facet)	**24**	Transverse process
12	Inferior vena cava	**25**	Zygapophysial (facet) joint
13	Intervertebral disc		

Lumbosacral spine, **(a)** sagittal MR image, **(b)** parasagittal MR image, **(c)** coronal STIR (short tau inversion recovery) MR image.

1	Annulus fibrosus	**12**	Interspinous ligament and bursa
2	Anterior longitudinal ligament	**13**	Intervertebral foramen
3	Basivertebral veins	**14**	Kidney
4	Body of third lumbar vertebra	**15**	Ligamentum flavum
5	Cauda equina	**16**	Nucleus pulposus
6	Caudal lumbar thecal sac	**17**	Pedicle
7	Cerebrospinal fluid	**18**	Posterior longitudinal ligament and annulus fibrosus
8	Conus medullaris	**19**	Psoas muscle
9	Epidural fat	**20**	Radicular vessels
10	Epidural space (fat filled)	**21**	Sacral promontory
11	Internuclear cleft	**22**	Spinal nerve root in intervertebral foramen

Cervical myelogram, **(a)** with the neck extended, **(b)** with the neck slightly flexed, anteroposterior projections.

Non-ionic water-soluble contrast medium is introduced into the lumbar subarachnoid space via a lumbar puncture. The patient is positioned prone, with the neck hyperextended, and strapped onto a tilting table. The contrast medium is then run up into the cervical region to demonstrate the cervical spinal cord and exiting nerve roots. There are eight cervical nerve roots: the roots of the eighth cervical nerve exit through the intervertebral foramina between the seventh cervical vertebra and the first thoracic vertebra. The normal cervical cord enlargement (3) (for the brachial plexus) extends from the third cervical vertebra to the second thoracic vertebra. It is maximal at the fifth cervical vertebra and should not be mistaken for an intramedullary lesion.

1 Anterior spinal artery
2 Cervical cord
3 Cervical cord enlargement
4 Cervical spinal nerve exiting through intervertebral foramen
5 Contrast medium in cervical subarachnoid space
6 Dorsal root of spinal nerve
7 First rib
8 Lateral mass of atlas (first cervical vertebra)
9 Normal large transverse process of seventh cervical vertebra
10 Occiput
11 Odontoid process (dens)
12 Root of eighth cervical nerve
13 Thoracic cord
14 Transverse foramen
15 Ventral root of spinal nerve
16 Vertebral artery

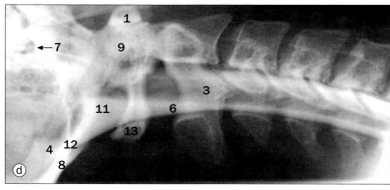

Cervical myelogram, **(c)** with the patient prone, **(d)** with the patient supine, lateral projections.

1 Anterior arch of atlas (first cervical vertebra)
2 Anterior rim of foramen magnum
3 Cervical cord
4 Cisterna magna (cerebellomedullary cistern)
5 Clivus
6 Contrast medium in cervical subarachnoid space
7 External acoustic meatus
8 Occiput
9 Odontoid (process) dens
10 Posterior indentation on theca from ligamentum flavum
11 Posterior inferior cerebellar artery
12 Posterior rim of foramen magnum
13 Posterior tubercle of atlas (first cervical vertebra)

Lumbar radiculogram, (a) lateral projection, (b) oblique projection, (c) anteroposterior projection.

Non-ionic water-soluble contrast medium is introduced into the lumbar subarachnoid space via a lumbar puncture. The nerve roots of the cauda equina are well demonstrated and exit through the intervertebral foramina. The nerve roots extending from the conus to the terminal thecal sac pass below the pedicle of the corresponding vertebra. The thecal sac terminates at the level of the first/second sacral vertebrae. The filum terminale may be seen. Tilting the prone patient slightly head down allows the contrast to flow cranially and outlines the conus and lower thoracic cord. The cord is uniform in size from the second to the tenth thoracic vertebra, at which point its second, smaller expansion (for the lumbosacral plexus) extends from the tenth thoracic vertebra to the level of the first lumbar vertebra. The conus medullaris usually terminates at the first/second lumbar vertebrae, but may be seen at a level above and below as a normal variant.

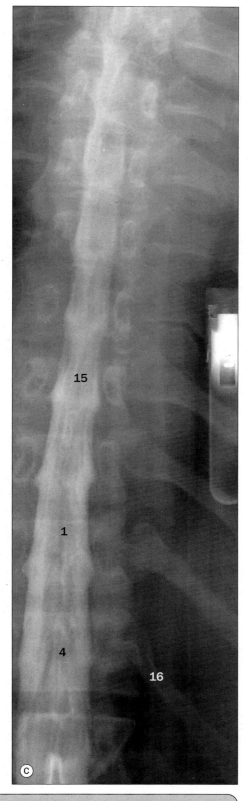

1	Anterior median fissure	
2	Body of second lumbar vertebra	
3	Contrast medium in subarachnoid space	
4	Conus medullaris	
5	Fifth lumbar spinal nerve	
6	Fourth lumbar spinal nerve	
7	Intervertebral disc indentations in anterior thecal margin	
8	Lateral extension of subarachnoid space around spinal nerve roots	
9	Lumbar puncture needle in space between third and fourth lumbar vertebrae	
10	Sacral promontory	
11	Spinal nerves within subarachnoid space (cauda equina)	
12	Spinous process of third lumbar vertebra	
13	Terminal theca at first/second sacral vertebra	
14	Test tube containing contrast medium to indicate tilt of patient	
15	Thoracic cord	
16	Twelfth rib	

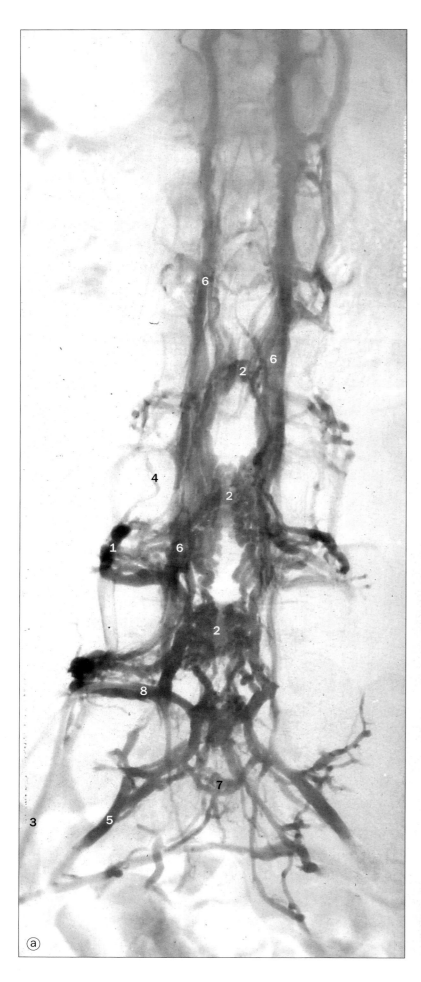

(a) Subtracted lumbar venogram.
Since the advent of CT and MR imaging techniques, lumbar venography is rarely performed. However, the anatomy of the vertebral veins is optimally demonstrated by this technique. Venous drainage of the spinal cord is longitudinally arranged via plexi, which anastomose freely with the internal (6) and external (1 and 4) vertebral venous plexi, which also communicate (4 and 2). Note how the internal veins bend laterally at the level of the disc interspace and medially at the level of pedicles, where they unite via a connecting vein (2).

1	Ascending lumbar veins
2	Basivertebral veins
3	Catheter in common iliac vein
4	Intervertebral veins
5	Lateral sacral veins
6	Longitudinal vertebral venous plexi
7	Sacral venous plexus
8	Tip of catheter in intravertebral vein

(b) Spinal arteriogram.

1	Anterior spinal artery
2	Arteria radicularis magna (Adamkiewicz)
3	Normal transdural stenosis of the arteria radicularis magna
4	Selective catheterisation of left eleventh intercostal artery

3 Upper limb

(a) Shoulder, anteroposterior radiograph.

1 Acromion of scapula
2 Anatomical neck
3 Clavicle
4 Coracoid process of scapula
5 Glenoid fossa of scapula
6 Greater tubercle (tuberosity) of humerus
7 Head of humerus
8 Intertubercular groove of humerus
9 Lesser tubercle (tuberosity) of humerus
10 Scapula
11 Surgical neck

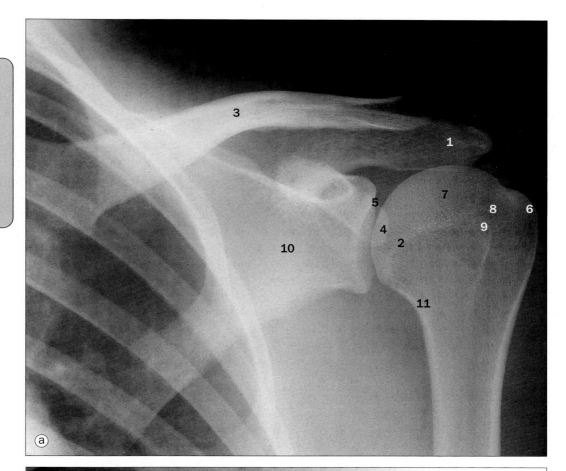

(b) Shoulder, axial (supero-inferior) projection.

1 Acromion of scapula
2 Clavicle
3 Coracoid process of scapula
4 Glenoid fossa of scapula
5 Greater tubercle (tuberosity) of humerus
6 Head of humerus
7 Intertubercular groove of humerus
8 Lesser tubercle (tuberosity) of humerus
9 Spine of scapula

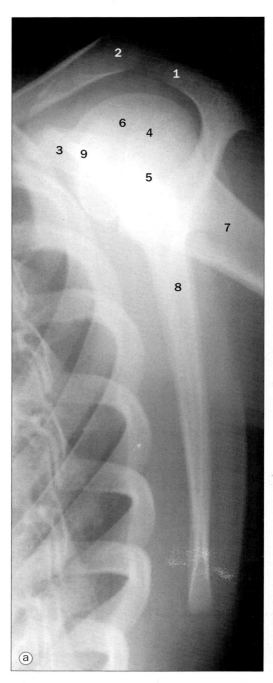

(a) Scapula of a 14-year-old boy, lateral projection.

Shoulder, **(b)** (anteroposterior) of a 1-year-old child, **(c)** (anteroposterior) and **(d)** (axial) of a 6-year-old child, **(e)** (anteroposterior) and **(f)** (axial) of a 14-year-old child.

1 Acromion of scapula
2 Centre for coracoid process
3 Centre for greater tubercle (tuberosity) of humerus
4 Centre for head of humerus
5 Clavicle
6 Epiphysial line
7 Glenoid fossa of scapula

1 Acromion
2 Clavicle
3 Coracoid process
4 Epiphysial line
5 Glenoid fossa
6 Head of humerus
7 Humerus
8 Lateral border of scapula
9 Spine of scapula

CLAVICLE (m)	Appears	Fused
Lateral end	5 wiu	20+ yrs
Medial end	15 yrs	20+ yrs
SCAPULA (c)		
Body	8 wiu	15 yrs
Coracoid	<1 yr	20 yrs
Coracoid base	Puberty	15–20 yrs
Acromion	Puberty	15–20 yrs

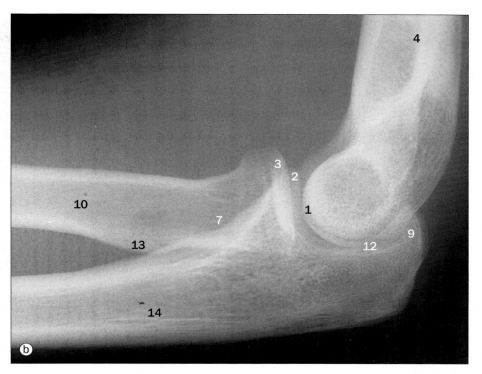

Elbow, (a) anteroposterior projection, (b) lateral projection, (c) axial projection.

1 Capitulum of humerus
2 Coronoid process of ulna
3 Head of radius
4 Humerus
5 Lateral epicondyle of humerus
6 Medial epicondyle of humerus
7 Neck of radius
8 Olecranon fossa of humerus
9 Olecranon of ulna
10 Radius
11 Trochlea of humerus
12 Trochlear notch of ulna
13 Tuberosity of radius
14 Ulna

HUMERUS (c)	Appears	Fused
Shaft	8 wiu	15–20 yrs
Head	1–6 mths	15–20 yrs
Greater tubercle	6 mths–1 yr	15–20 yrs
Lesser tubercle	3–5 yrs	18–20 yrs
Capitulum	4 mths–1 yr	13–16 yrs
Medial trochlea	10 yrs	13–16 yrs
Medial epicondyle	3–6 yrs	13–16 yrs
Lateral epicondyle	9–12 yrs	13–16 yrs
RADIUS (c)		
Shaft	8 wiu	
Proximal	4–6 yrs	13–16 yrs
Distal	1 yr	16–18 yrs
ULNA (c)		
Shaft	8 wiu	
Proximal	8–10 yrs	13–15 yrs
Distal	5–7 yrs	16–18 yrs

Elbow, (**a**) (anteroposterior) of a 1-year-old child, (**b**) (lateral) and (**c**) (anteroposterior) of a 3-year-old child, (**d**) (anteroposterior) of a 6-year-old child, (**e**) (anteroposterior) of a 9-year-old child, (**f**) (lateral) of an 11-year-old child, (**g**) (lateral) and (**h**) (anteroposterior) of a 14-year-old child, to illustrate centres of ossification.

1 Centre for capitulum
2 Centre for lateral epicondyle
3 Centre for medial epicondyle
4 Centre for olecranon
5 Centre for radial head
6 Centre for trochlea
7 Epiphysial line
8 Humerus
9 Radius
10 Ulna

1 Base of fifth metacarpal
2 Base of middle phalanx of middle finger
3 Base of proximal phalanx of ring finger
4 Capitate
5 Distal phalanx of index finger
6 Distal phalanx of thumb
7 Hamate
8 Head of fifth metacarpal
9 Head of middle phalanx of middle finger
10 Head of ulna
11 Head proximal phalanx of ring finger
12 Hook of hamate
13 Lunate
14 Middle phalanx of index finger
15 Pisiform
16 Proximal phalanx of index finger
17 Proximal phalanx of thumb
18 Radius
19 Scaphoid
20 Second metacarpal
21 Sesamoid bone
22 Shaft of fifth metacarpal
23 Shaft of middle phalanx of middle finger
24 Shaft of proximal phalanx of ring finger
25 Styloid process of radius
26 Styloid process of ulna
27 Trapezium
28 Trapezoid
29 Triquetral
30 Ulnar notch of radius

• There are often two sesamoids (21), present in the flexor pollicis brevis and adductor pollicis muscles.

(a) Bones of the hand, dorsopalmar projection.

(b) Bones of the wrist, lateral projection.

Bones of the hand (dorsopalmar projections), (**a**) of a 3-month-old boy, (**b**) of a 3-year-old boy, (**c**) of a 6-year-old boy, (**d**) of an 11-year-old boy, to illustrate centres of ossification.

CARPUS (c)	Appears	Fused
Capitate	1–3 mths	
Hamate	2–4 mths	
Triquetral	2–3 yrs	
Lunate	2–4 yrs	
Scaphoid	4–6 yrs	
Trapezium	4–6 yrs	
Trapezoid	4–6 yrs	
Pisiform (sesamoid)	8–12 yrs	
METACARPALS (c)		
Shaft	9 wiu	
Head	1–2 yrs	14–19 yrs
PHALANGES (c)		
Shaft	8–12 wiu	
Base	1–3 yrs	14–18 yrs

1 Capitate
2 Centre for distal phalanx of middle finger
3 Centre for distal radius
4 Centre for distal ulna
5 Centre for first metacarpal
6 Centre for middle phalanx of middle finger
7 Centre for proximal phalanx of middle finger
8 Centre for second metacarpal (applies to second to fifth metacarpals)
9 Epiphysial line
10 Hamate
11 Lunate
12 Radius
13 Scaphoid
14 Trapezium
15 Trapezoid
16 Triquetral
17 Ulna

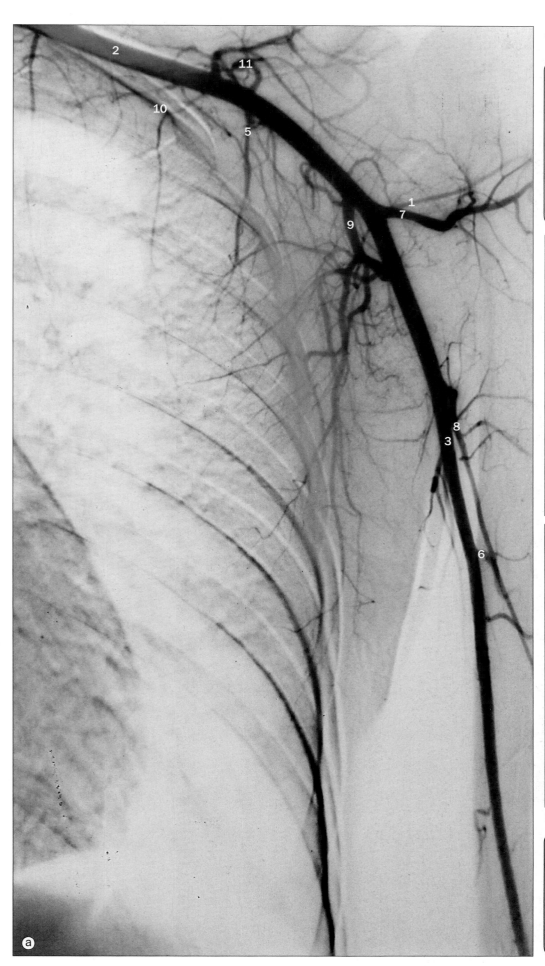

Axillary arteriograms, (a) subtracted,
(b) digitally subtracted.

1	Anterior circumflex humeral artery
2	Axillary artery
3	Brachial artery
4	Circumflex scapular artery
5	Lateral thoracic artery
6	Muscular branches of brachial artery
7	Posterior circumflex humeral artery
8	Profunda brachii artery
9	Subscapular artery
10	Superior thoracic artery
11	Thoraco-acromial artery

(c) Superior vena cavogram, subtracted.

1	Axillary vein
2	Basilic vein
3	Brachiocephalic vein
4	Cephalic vein
5	Right atrium
6	Site of entry of left brachiocephalic vein
7	Subclavian vein
8	Superior vena cava

Brachial arteriogram.

1	Anterior interosseous artery
2	Brachial artery
3	Common interosseous artery
4	Posterior interosseous artery
5	Radial artery
6	Radial recurrent artery
7	Ulnar artery
8	Ulnar recurrent artery

(a) Digitally subtracted hand arteriogram.
In this patient there is an incomplete superficial palmar arch.

(b) Venous phase of hand arteriogram.

1	Artery to radial aspects of thumb
2	Common palmar digital artery
3	Deep palmar arch
4	Deep palmar branch of ulnar artery
5	Palmar carpal branch of ulnar artery
6	Palmar metacarpal artery
7	Princeps pollicis artery
8	Proper palmar digital artery
9	Radial artery
10	Ulnar artery

1	Basilic vein
2	Cephalic vein
3	Common palmar digital vein
4	Palmar digital vein
5	Princeps pollicis vein
6	Radialis indicis vein
7	Superficial palmar venous arch

Shoulder, axial MR images, (a)–(f) axial images, (g)–(l) oblique sagittal images.

1 Acromioclavicular joint	**9** Clavicle	**17** Glenoid labrum
2 Acromion	**10** Coracobrachialis muscle	**18** Greater tuberosity
3 Anterior capsule of shoulder joint	**11** Coracoclavicular ligament	**19** Head of humerus
4 Anterior labrum	**12** Coracohumeral ligament	**20** Humerus
5 Axillary artery and vein	**13** Coracoid process	**21** Inferior glenohumeral ligament
6 Axillary recess	**14** Deltoid tendon	**22** Inferior labrum
7 Biceps brachii tendon	**15** Deltoid muscle	**23** Infraspinatus muscle
8 Biceps brachii tendon - long head	**16** Glenoid	**24** Infraspinatus tendon

25 Middle glenohumeral ligament	**30** Scapula	**35** Superior labrum
26 Pectoralis minor muscle	**31** Spine of scapula	**36** Supraspinatus muscle
27 Posterior capsule of shoulder joint	**32** Subscapularis muscle	**37** Supraspinatus tendon
28 Posterior labrum	**33** Subscapularis tendon	**38** Teres minor muscle
29 Rotator cuff	**34** Superior glenohumeral ligament	**39** Trapezius muscle

(a)–(f) Shoulder, coronal oblique MR images. See pages 74 and 75 for key.

Post gadolinium arthrogram, MR images. **(a)**–**(d)** Sagittal oblique projection, **(e)**–**(h)** axial projection, **(i)**–**(l)** coronal oblique projection. See pages 74 and 75 for key.

Post gadolinium arthrogram, MR images. (g) and (h) axial projection, (i)–(l) coronal oblique projection.
See pages 74 and 75 for key.

(a)–(d) Elbow, sagittal MR images.

1 Abductor pollicis longus muscle
2 Anterior fat pad
3 Biceps brachii muscle
4 Biceps brachii tendon
5 Brachial artery
6 Brachialis muscle
7 Brachioradialis muscle
8 Capitulum of humerus
9 Cephalic vein
10 Coronoid process of ulna
11 Flexor carpi ulnaris muscle
12 Flexor digitorum profundus muscle
13 Flexor digitorum superficialis muscle
14 Head of radius
15 Humerus
16 Lateral head of triceps muscle
17 Medial epicondyle
18 Medial head of triceps muscle
19 Olecranon fossa of humerus
20 Olecranon process of ulna
21 Pronator teres muscle
22 Radius
23 Supinator muscle
24 Tendon of triceps muscle
25 Trochlea of humerus

(a)–(d) Elbow, coronal MR images.

1	Basilic vein
2	Biceps brachii muscle
3	Brachial artery
4	Brachialis muscle
5	Brachioradialis muscle
6	Capitulum of humerus
7	Cephalic vein
8	Common extensor origin
9	Common flexor origin
10	Extensor carpi radialis brevis muscle
11	Extensor carpi radialis longus muscle
12	Flexor carpi radialis muscle
13	Flexor carpi ulnaris muscle
14	Flexor digitorum profundus muscle
15	Flexor digitorum superficialis muscle
16	Head of radius
17	Humerus
18	Lateral epicondyle
19	Lateral head of triceps muscle
20	Lateral supracondylar ridge
21	Long head of triceps muscle
22	Medial epicondyle
23	Medial head of triceps muscle
24	Medial supracondylar ridge
25	Olecranon fossa of humerus
26	Olecranon process of ulna
27	Pronator teres muscle
28	Radius
29	Supinator muscle
30	Tendon of biceps brachii muscle
31	Trochlea of humerus
32	Tuberosity of radius
33	Ulna

(a)–(e) Elbow, axial MR images.

1	Anconeus muscle	**20**	Lateral epicondyle
2	Basilic vein	**21**	Lateral head of triceps muscle
3	Biceps brachii muscle	**22**	Lateral supracondylar ridge
4	Bicipital aponeurosis	**23**	Long head of triceps muscle
5	Brachial artery	**24**	Medial epicondyle
6	Brachialis muscle	**25**	Medial head of triceps muscle
7	Brachialis tendon	**26**	Medial supracondylar ridge
8	Brachioradialis muscle	**27**	Median nerve
9	Cephalic vein	**28**	Olecranon fossa of humerus
10	Common extensor origin	**29**	Olecranon process of ulna
11	Common flexor origin	**30**	Palmaris longus muscle
12	Extensor carpi radialis brevis muscle	**31**	Profunda brachii artery
13	Extensor carpi radialis longus muscle	**32**	Pronator teres muscle
14	Flexor carpi radialis muscle	**33**	Radial artery
15	Flexor carpi ulnaris muscle	**34**	Radial nerve
16	Flexor digitorum profundus muscle	**35**	Radius
17	Flexor digitorum superficialis muscle	**36**	Supinator muscle
18	Head of radius	**37**	Tendon of biceps brachii muscle
19	Humerus	**38**	Ulna
		39	Ulnar nerve

(a)–(d) Forearm, axial MR images.

1	Abductor pollicis longus muscle	**15**	Flexor digitorum profundus muscle
2	Anconeus muscle	**16**	Flexor digitorum superficialis muscle
3	Anterior interosseous artery	**17**	Interosseous membrane
4	Basilic vein	**18**	Median nerve
5	Brachioradialis muscle	**19**	Palmaris longus muscle
6	Cephalic vein	**20**	Pronator teres muscle
7	Extensor carpi radialis brevis muscle	**21**	Radial artery
8	Extensor carpi radialis longus muscle	**22**	Radial nerve
9	Extensor carpi radialis longus tendon	**23**	Radius
10	Extensor carpi ulnaris muscle	**24**	Supinator muscle
11	Extensor digitorum muscle	**25**	Ulna
12	Extensor pollicis longus muscle	**26**	Ulnar artery
13	Flexor carpi radialis muscle	**27**	Ulnar nerve
14	Flexor carpi ulnaris muscle		

(a)–(e) Wrist, axial MR images.

1 Abductor digiti minimi muscle	**21** Tendon of abductor pollicis longus muscle
2 Abductor pollicis brevis muscle	**22** Tendon of extensor carpi radialis brevis muscle
3 Base of first metacarpal	**23** Tendon of extensor carpi radialis longus muscle
4 Basilic vein	**24** Tendon of extensor carpi ulnaris muscle
5 Capitate	**25** Tendon of extensor digiti minimi muscle
6 Cephalic vein	**26** Tendon of extensor digitorum muscle
7 Dorsal tubercle of radius	**27** Tendon of extensor pollicis brevis muscle
8 Dorsal venous arch	**28** Tendon of extensor pollicis longus muscle
9 Flexor digitorum superficialis muscle	**29** Tendon of flexor carpi radialis muscle
10 Flexor retinaculum	**30** Tendon of flexor carpi ulnaris muscle
11 Guyon's canal	**31** Tendon of flexor digitorum profundus muscle
12 Hamate	**32** Tendon of flexor digitorum superficialis muscle
13 Hook of hamate	**33** Tendon of flexor pollicis longus muscle
14 Lunate	**34** Tendon of palmaris longus muscle
15 Median nerve	**35** Trapezium
16 Pisiform	**36** Trapezoid
17 Radial artery	**37** Triquetral
18 Radius	**38** Ulna
19 Scaphoid	**39** Ulnar artery
20 Styloid process of ulna	**40** Ulnar nerve

(a)–(e) Hand, axial MR images.

1 Abductor digiti minimi muscle	**19** Proximal phalanx of index finger
2 Abductor pollicis brevis muscle	**20** Superficial palmar arch
3 Adductor pollicis muscle	**21** Tendon of extensor digiti
4 Base of first metacarpal	minimi muscle
5 Base of fourth metacarpal	**22** Tendon of extensor digitorum
6 Base of second metacarpal	muscle
7 Base of third metacarpal	**23** Tendon of extensor pollicis
8 Distal phalanx of thumb	brevis muscle
9 Dorsal interossei muscles	**24** Tendon of extensor pollicis
10 Flexor digiti minimi muscle	longus muscle
11 Flexor pollicis brevis muscle	**25** Tendon of flexor digitorum
12 Head of fifth metacarpal	profundus muscle
13 Head of first metacarpal	**26** Tendon of flexor digitorum
14 Lumbrical muscle	superficialis muscle
15 Metacarpal shaft	**27** Tendon of flexor pollicis longus
16 Opponens digiti minimi muscle	muscle
17 Opponens pollicis muscle	**28** Ulnar artery
18 Palmar interossei muscles	

(a)–(d) Hand, coronal MR images.

1	Abductor digiti minimi muscle	**15**	Lumbrical muscle
2	Abductor pollicis brevis muscle	**16**	Middle phalanx
3	Adductor pollicis muscle	**17**	Opponens digiti minimi muscle
4	Base of proximal phalanx	**18**	Opponens pollicis muscle
5	Capitate	**19**	Palmar interossei muscles
6	Common palmar digital artery	**20**	Proper palmar digital artery
7	Deep palmar arch	**21**	Proximal phalanx of thumb
8	Distal phalanx of thumb	**22**	Shaft of proximal phalanx
9	Dorsal interossei muscles	**23**	Tendon of extensor pollicis longus muscle
10	Flexor digiti minimi muscle	**24**	Tendon of flexor digitorum profundus muscle
11	Flexor pollicis brevis muscle	**25**	Tendon of flexor digitorum superficialis muscle
12	Hamate	**26**	Tendon of flexor pollicis longus muscle
13	Head of fifth metacarpal	**27**	Trapezium
14	Head of first metacarpal	**28**	Trapezoid

4 Thorax

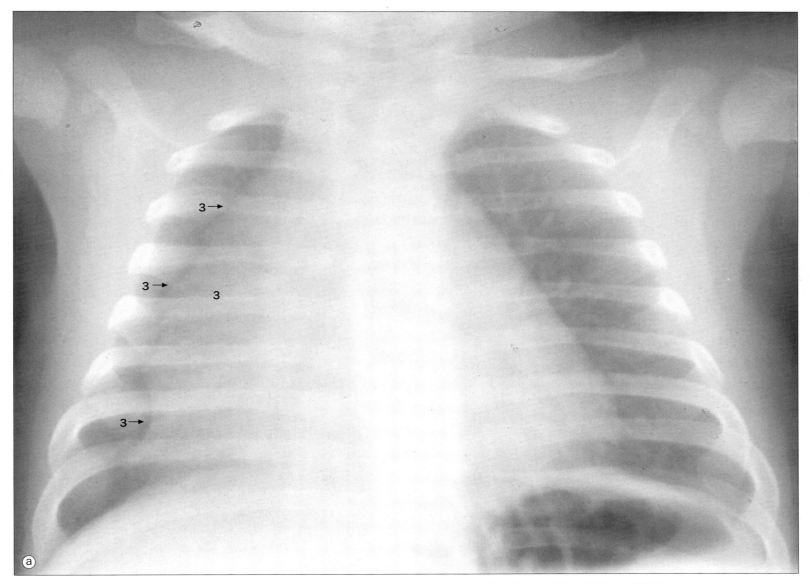

(a) Chest of a 4-month-old child, postero-anterior radiograph.
(b) Cervical rib, adult, postero-anterior projection.
(c) Azygos fissure, adult, postero-anterior projection.

1	Azygos fissure
2	Cervical rib
3	Thymus

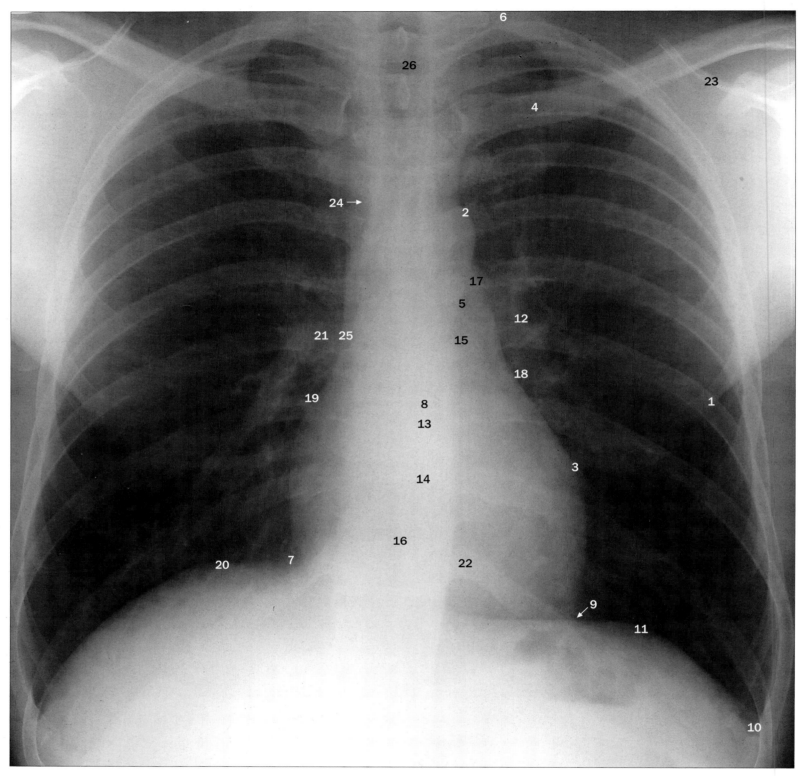

Chest of an adult male, postero-anterior projection.

1 Anterior axillary fold	**10** Left costophrenic angle	**19** Right atrial border
2 Arch of aorta (aortic knuckle or knob)	**11** Left dome of diaphragm	**20** Right dome of diaphragm
3 Border of left ventricle	**12** Left pulmonary artery	**21** Right pulmonary artery
4 Clavicle	**13** Position of aortic valve	**22** Right ventricle
5 Descending aorta	**14** Position of mitral valve	**23** Spine of scapula
6 First rib	**15** Position of pulmonary valve	**24** Sternum
7 Inferior vena cava	**16** Position of tricuspid valve	**25** Superior vena cava
8 Left atrium	**17** Pulmonary trunk	**26** Trachea
9 Left cardiophrenic angle	**18** Region of tip of auricle of left atrium	

Chest of an adult female, lateral projection.

1 Arch of aorta (aortic knuckle or knob)	**9** Left dome of diaphragm	**18** Right main bronchus
2 Ascending aorta	**10** Left main bronchus	**19** Right main pulmonary artery
3 Breast	**11** Left main pulmonary artery	**20** Right ventricle
4 Gas in fundus of stomach	**12** Left oblique fissure	**21** Right ventricular border of heart
5 Inferior vena cava	**13** Position of aortic valve	**22** Scapula
6 Infundibulum of right ventricle (below) with	**14** Position of mitral valve	**23** Soft tissues of upper arm
pulmonary trunk (above)	**15** Position of pulmonary valve	**24** Trachea
7 Left atrial border of heart	**16** Position of tricuspid valve	
8 Left atrium	**17** Right dome of diaphragm	

1	Inframammary fold
2	Lactiferous duct
3	Lactiferous sinus
4	Line of skin
5	Lobar duct pattern (comprising (intra) lobar ducts and terminal ductal lobular units)
6	Mammary fat
7	Mammary fibroglandular tissue
8	Nipple
9	Pectoral muscle
10	Subareolar area
11	Suspensory ligament (Cooper's)

(a) Postmenopausal right breast, medio–lateral oblique mammogram.

(b) Premenopausal left breast, lateral oblique mammogram.

(c) Premenopausal right breast, craniocaudal image from a ductogram.

(d) Mammogram, MR image.

(a)–(l) Chest, CT images of mediastinum.

1 Arch of aorta (aortic knuckle or knob)	**19** Oesophagus
2 Body of sternum	**20** Pectoralis major muscle
3 Body of vertebra	**21** Pectoralis minor muscle
4 Brachial plexus	**22** Pedicle
5 Brachiocephalic trunk	**23** Right brachiocephalic vein
6 Clavicle	**24** Right subclavian artery
7 Costotransverse joint	**25** Right subclavian vein
8 Costovertebral joint	**26** Serratus anterior muscle
9 Erector spinae muscle	**27** Spinal cord
10 Head of rib	**28** Sternoclavicular joint
11 Infraspinatus muscle	**29** Sternocleidomastoid muscle
12 Intervertebral foramen	**30** Subscapularis muscle
13 Lamina	**31** Superior vena cava
14 Latissimus dorsi muscle	**32** Supraspinatus muscle
15 Left brachiocephalic vein	**33** Teres major muscle
16 Left common carotid artery	**34** Trachea
17 Left subclavian artery	**35** Transverse process
18 Manubrium of sternum	**36** Trapezius muscle

(e)–(h) Chest, CT images of mediastinum.

1 Anterior interventricular branch of left coronary artery	**14** Infraspinatus muscle
2 Ascending aorta	**15** Internal thoracic artery and vein
3 Azygos vein	**16** Lamina
4 Body of sternum	**17** Latissimus dorsi muscle
5 Body of vertebra	**18** Left atrial appendage (auricle)
6 Carina (bifurcation of trachea)	**19** Left atrium
7 Coronary sinus	**20** Left inferior lobe bronchus
8 Costotransverse joint	**21** Left inferior pulmonary vein
9 Descending aorta	**22** Left main bronchus
10 Erector spinae muscle	**23** Left pulmonary artery
11 Head of rib	**24** Left superior lobe bronchus
12 Hemi-azygos vein	**25** Left superior pulmonary vein
13 Inferior vena cava	**26** Left ventricular cavity

(i)–(l) Chest, CT images of mediastinum.

27 Oesophagus	41 Right superior pulmonary vein
28 Pectoralis major muscle	42 Right ventricular cavity
29 Pectoralis minor muscle	43 Serratus anterior muscle
30 Pedicle	44 Spinal cord
31 Pericardium	45 Subscapularis muscle
32 Pulmonary trunk	46 Superior lobe branch of right pulmonary artery
33 Rhomboid major muscle	47 Superior pericardial recess
34 Right atrial appendage (auricle)	48 Superior vena cava
35 Right atrium	49 Teres major muscle
36 Right inferior lobe bronchus	50 Teres minor muscle
37 Right inferior pulmonary vein	51 Trachea
38 Right main bronchus	52 Transverse process
39 Right pulmonary artery	53 Trapezius muscle
40 Right superior lobe bronchus	

(a)–(h) Lungs, axial high resolution CT images.

1 Anterior segment superior lobe	**11** Horizontal fissure
2 Anterior segmental bronchus	**12** Lateral segment middle lobe
3 Aorta	**13** Left brachiocephalic vein
4 Apical segment inferior lobe	**14** Left common carotid artery
5 Apical segment right superior lobe	**15** Left inferior lobe bronchus
6 Apicoposterior segment left superior lobe	**16** Left main bronchus
7 Azygos arch	**17** Left subclavian artery
8 Azygos vein	**18** Left superior lobe bronchus
9 Brachiocephalic trunk	**19** Left superior pulmonary vein
10 Bronchus intermedius	**20** Lingular segmental bronchus

21 Manubrium of sternum	**29** Right main bronchus
22 Medial segment middle lobe	**30** Right superior lobe bronchus
23 Oblique fissure	**31** Sternum
24 Oesophagus	**32** Superior lingular segment
25 Posterior segment superior lobe	**33** Superior pericardial recess
26 Posterior segmental bronchus	**34** Superior vena cava
27 Pulmonary artery	**35** Trachea
28 Right brachiocephalic vein	

(i)–(p) Lungs, axial high resolution CT images.

1 Anterior basal segment inferior lobe	10 Inferior lingular segment
2 Anterior basal segmental bronchus	11 Inferior lingular segmental bronchus
3 Anterior segment superior lobe	12 Inferior vena cava
4 Aorta	13 Lateral basal segment inferior lobe
5 Apical segment inferior lobe bronchus	14 Lateral basal segmental bronchus
6 Azygos vein	15 Lateral segment middle lobe
7 Heart	16 Lateral segmental bronchus of middle lobe
8 Hemi-azygos vein	17 Left inferior lobe bronchus
9 Horizontal fissure	

18 Liver	26 Posterior basal segmental bronchus
19 Medial basal segment inferior lobe	27 Right inferior lobe bronchus
20 Medial basal segmental bronchus	28 Right inferior pulmonary vein
21 Medial segment middle lobe	29 Right lower lobe pulmonary artery
22 Medial segmental bronchus of middle lobe	30 Spleen
23 Middle lobe bronchus	31 Stomach
24 Oblique fissure	32 Superior lingular segment
25 Posterior basal segment inferior lobe	33 Superior lingular segmental bronchus

(a)–(l) Chest, axial MR images.

1 Anterior interventricular branch of left coronary artery	**18** Interatrial septum
2 Arch of aorta (aortic knuckle or knob)	**19** Intercostal artery
3 Ascending aorta	**20** Internal thoracic artery and vein
4 Axillary artery	**21** Left atrial appendage (auricle)
5 Axillary vein	**22** Left atrium
6 Azygos vein	**23** Left brachiocephalic vein
7 Body of sternum	**24** Left common carotid artery
8 Body of vertebra	**25** Left coronary artery
9 Brachial plexus	**26** Left inferior lobe bronchus
10 Brachiocephalic trunk	**27** Left inferior pulmonary vein
11 Carina (bifurcation of trachea)	**28** Left main bronchus
12 Circumflex branch of left coronary artery	**29** Left pulmonary artery
13 Clavicle	**30** Left subclavian artery
14 Descending aorta	**31** Left superior intercostal vein
15 Erector spinae muscle	**32** Left superior lobe bronchus
16 Hemi-azygos vein	**33** Left superior pulmonary vein
17 Inferior vena cava	

34 Left ventricular cavity	**50** Right inferior lobe bronchus
35 Manubrium of sternum	**51** Right inferior pulmonary vein
36 Membranous interventricular septum	**52** Right main bronchus
37 Mitral valve	**53** Right pulmonary artery
38 Muscular interventricular septum	**54** Right superior intercostal vein
39 Oesophagus	**55** Right superior lobe bronchus
40 Papillary muscles	**56** Right superior pulmonary vein
41 Pectoralis major muscle	**57** Right ventricular cavity
42 Pectoralis minor muscle	**58** Serratus anterior muscle
43 Pericardial recess	**59** Sternoclavicular joint
44 Pericardium	**60** Subscapularis muscle
45 Pulmonary trunk	**61** Superior lobe branch of right pulmonary artery
46 Right atrial appendage (auricle)	**62** Superior vena cava
47 Right atrium	**63** Trachea
48 Right brachiocephalic vein	**64** Trapezius muscle
49 Right coronary artery	**65** Tricuspid valve

(a)–(f) Chest, coronal MR images.

1 Arch of aorta (aortic knuckle or knob)	26 Membranous interventricular septum
2 Ascending aorta	27 Muscular interventricular septum
3 Axillary artery	28 Papillary muscle
4 Axillary vein	29 Pulmonary trunk
5 Azygos vein	30 Right atrium
6 Body of vertebra	31 Right brachiocephalic vein
7 Brachial plexus	32 Right common carotid artery
8 Brachiocephalic trunk	33 Right inferior lobe bronchus
9 Carina (bifurcation of trachea)	34 Right main bronchus
10 Clavicle	35 Right pulmonary artery
11 Descending aorta	36 Right subclavian artery
12 Inferior vena cava	37 Right superior lobe bronchus
13 Infraspinatus muscle	38 Right superior pulmonary vein
14 Interatrial septum	39 Right ventricular cavity
15 Latissimus dorsi muscle	40 Right ventricular wall
16 Left atrial appendage (auricle)	41 Serratus anterior muscle
17 Left atrium	42 Sternocleidomastoid muscle
18 Left brachiocephalic vein	43 Subscapularis muscle
19 Left common carotid artery	44 Superior vena cava
20 Left main bronchus	45 Supraspinatus muscle
21 Left pulmonary artery	46 Teres major muscle
22 Left subclavian artery	47 Teres minor muscle
23 Left superior pulmonary vein	48 Trachea
24 Left ventricular cavity	49 Trapezius muscle
25 Left ventricular wall	

(a)–(f) Chest, sagittal MR images.

1 Arch of aorta (aortic knuckle or knob)	**21** Left ventricular cavity
2 Ascending aorta	**22** Manubrium of sternum
3 Body of sternum	**23** Muscular interventricular septum
4 Body of vertebra	**24** Oesophagus
5 Brachiocephalic trunk	**25** Pericardium
6 Clavicle	**26** Pulmonary trunk
7 Cusp (leaflet) of mitral valve	**27** Right atrium
8 Descending aorta	**28** Right common carotid artery
9 Fossa ovalis	**29** Right inferior pulmonary vein
10 Inferior vena cava	**30** Right main bronchus
11 Interatrial septum	**31** Right pulmonary artery
12 Internal jugular vein	**32** Right ventricular cavity
13 Left atrium	**33** Right ventricular wall
14 Left brachiocephalic vein	**34** Spinal cord
15 Left common carotid artery	**35** Sternoclavicular joint
16 Left inferior pulmonary vein	**36** Sternocleidomastoid muscle
17 Left main bronchus	**37** Superior vena cava
18 Left pulmonary artery	**38** Thyroid lobe
19 Left subclavian artery	**39** Trachea
20 Left superior pulmonary vein	**40** Vertebral artery

Pulmonary arteriogram, arterial phase.

1 Anterior artery (superior lobe)	**10** Medial artery (middle lobe)
2 Anterior basal artery	**11** Medial basal artery
3 Apical artery (superior lobe)	**12** Middle lobe pulmonary artery
4 Catheter introduced via right brachial vein	**13** Posterior artery (superior lobe)
5 Inferior lingular artery	**14** Posterior basal artery
6 Inferior lobe pulmonary artery	**15** Right pulmonary artery
7 Lateral artery (middle lobe)	**16** Superior lingular artery
8 Lateral basal artery	**17** Superior lobe pulmonary artery
9 Left pulmonary artery	**18** Tip of catheter in main pulmonary artery

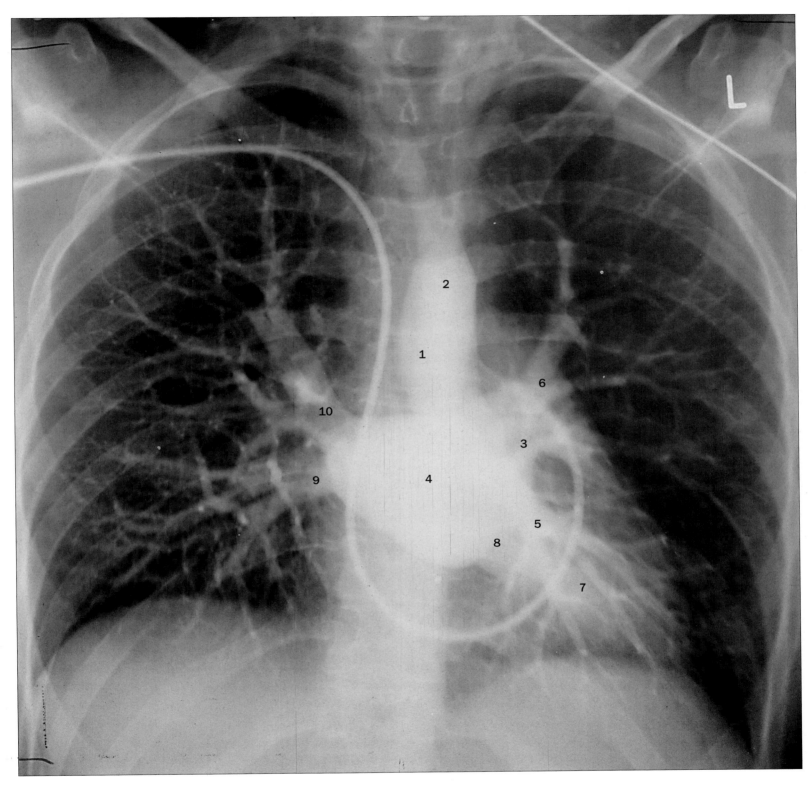

Pulmonary arteriogram – venous phase.

1 Aorta	**6** Left superior pulmonary vein
2 Aortic arch	**7** Left ventricle
3 Left atrial appendage (auricle)	**8** Mitral valve
4 Left atrium	**9** Right inferior pulmonary vein
5 Left inferior pulmonary vein	**10** Right superior pulmonary vein

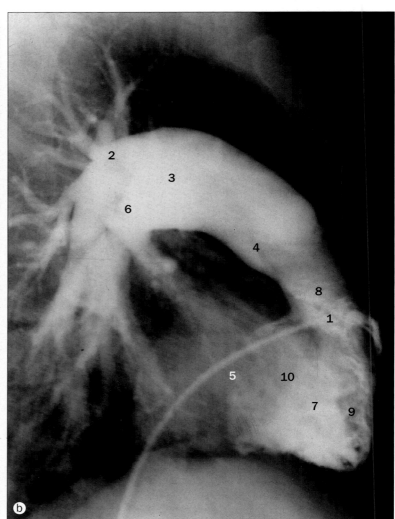

(a) and (b) Right ventricular angiograms.

1   Catheter in right ventricle via inferior vena cava and right atrium
2   Left main pulmonary artery
3   Pulmonary artery
4   Pulmonary valve
5   Right atrium
6   Right main pulmonary artery
7   Right ventricle
8   Right ventricular outflow tract
9   Trabeculae of right ventricle
10 Tricuspid valve

(a) Left coronary arteriogram, (b) right coronary arteriogram, (c) left ventricular angiogram, diastolic phase, (d) left ventricular angiogram, systolic phase.

1 Aorta	**10** First obtuse marginal branch of circumflex artery	**16** Left main stem coronary artery
2 Aortic sinus	**11** Inferior wall of left ventricle	**17** Left ventricular cavity
3 Aortic valve	**12** Lateral ventricular branch to left ventricle	**18** Left ventricular outflow tract
4 Apex of the left ventricle	**13** Left anterior interventricular artery curving round apex of heart	**19** Mitral valve
5 Atrioventricular nodal artery	**14** Left anterior interventricular branch (left anterior descending)	**20** Posterior interventricular septal artery (posterior descending artery)
6 Branch to left atrium	**15** Left coronary artery	**21** Right coronary artery
7 Circumflex artery		**22** Right marginal arteries
8 Conus artery		**23** Septal arteries
9 Diagonal arteries		**24** Sinuatrial nodal artery

Heart, **(a)** suprasternal arch of aorta, **(b)** left parasternal long axis of left ventricle, **(c)** left parasternal short axis at aortic valve, **(d)** left parasternal short axis at papillary muscles, **(e)** apical four chamber, **(f)** subcostal four chamber. Ultrasound images.

1 Anterior leaflet of the mitral valve	**9** Descending aorta	**18** Left subclavian artery	**27** Pulmonary valve
2 Anterior wall of right ventricle	**10** Inferior wall of left ventricle	**19** Left ventricle	**28** Pulmonary vein
3 Aorta	**11** Interatrial septum	**20** Left ventricular cavity	**29** Right atrium
4 Aortic sinus	**12** Interventricular septum	**21** Left ventricular outflow tract	**30** Right ventricle
5 Aortic valve	**13** Left atrium	**22** Mitral valve	**31** Right ventricular cavity
6 Ascending aorta	**14** Left common carotid artery	**23** Myocardium	**32** Right ventricular outflow tract
7 Brachiocephalic trunk	**15** Left coronary artery	**24** Papillary muscles	**33** Tricuspid valve
8 Chordae tendineae	**16** Left lobe of liver	**25** Pericardium	
	17 Left pulmonary artery	**26** Posterior leaflet of the mitral valve	

(a) Subtracted arch aortagram, anteroposterior image.
• The vertebral artery (22) has a separate origin off the arch, projected over the left common carotid artery in this view. This is a normal variant.

(b) Subtracted arch aortogram, left anterior oblique image.
The origins of the supra-aortic branches are best shown by left anterior oblique projection, so that the origins of the vessels are not superimposed. There are many congenital variations in the way in which the major vessels arise from the aortic arch, but the most common is shown in (b).

(c) Arch aortogram.

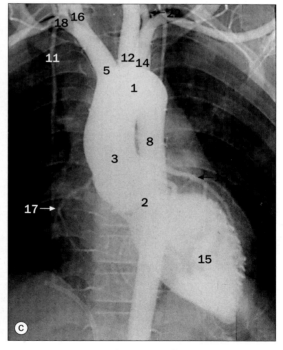

1	Aortic arch	12	Left common carotid artery
2	Aortic valve	13	Left coronary artery
3	Ascending aorta	14	Left subclavian artery
4	Ascending cervical artery	15	Left ventricle
5	Brachiocephalic trunk	16	Right common carotid artery
6	Costocervical trunk	17	Right coronary artery
7	Deltoid branch of thoraco-acromial artery	18	Right subclavian artery
		19	Superior thoracic artery
8	Descending aorta	20	Suprascapular artery
9	Inferior thyroid artery	21	Thyrocervical trunk
10	Intercostal artery	22	Vertebral artery
11	Internal thoracic artery		

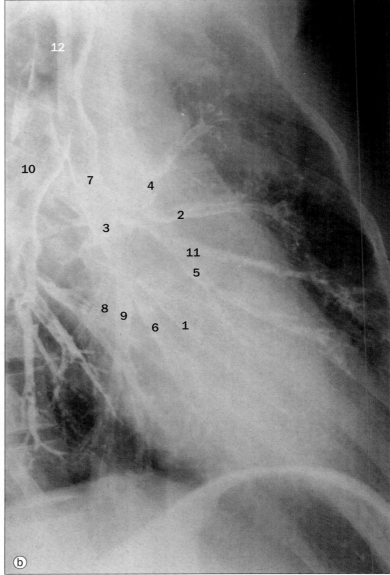

Left lung bronchogram, (a) postero-anterior image,
(b) oblique projection.

 1 Anterior basal segmental bronchus
 2 Anterior segmental bronchus
 3 Apical (superior) segmental bronchus
 4 Apicoposterior segmental bronchus
 5 Inferior lingular segmental bronchus
 6 Lateral basal segmental bronchus
 7 Left main bronchus
 8 Medial basal segmental bronchus
 9 Posterior basal segmental bronchus
10 Right main bronchus
11 Superior lingular segmental bronchus
12 Trachea

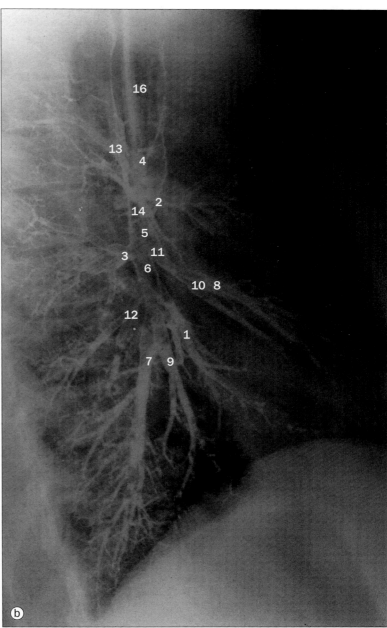

Right lung bronchogram, (a) postero-anterior projection, (b) lateral projection.

1 Anterior basal segmental bronchus	9 Medial basal segmental bronchus
2 Anterior segmental bronchus	10 Medial segmental bronchus of middle lobe
3 Apical (superior) segmental bronchus	11 Middle lobe bronchus
4 Apical segmental bronchus	12 Posterior basal segmental bronchus
5 Bronchus intermedius	13 Posterior segmental bronchus
6 Inferior lobe bronchus	14 Right main bronchus
7 Lateral basal segmental bronchus	15 Right superior lobe bronchus
8 Lateral segmental bronchus of middle lobe	16 Trachea

(a)–(c) Right bronchial arteriograms.

There is a great variability in the anatomy of the bronchial arteries, but the majority originate from the descending thoracic aorta, above the level of the left main stem bronchus between the upper border of the fifth thoracic vertebra and the lower border of the sixth thoracic vertebra. The number of bronchial arteries on each side may vary between one and four. Usually, there is one vessel to the right lung and two to the left. Accessory bronchial arteries may arise from the brachiocephalic artery and subclavian arteries, or from other branches such as the internal thoracic, pericardiophrenic and oesophageal arteries. In many cases the right bronchial artery arises from an intercostobronchial trunk, but in this example the trunk is very short and divides almost immediately into a right bronchial artery, which is directed towards the hilum, and the first right aortic intercostal artery. Reflux filling of the left bronchial artery is seen.
 A second larger bronchial artery which has been catheterised **(b)** has a common trunk arising from the front of the aorta, giving rise to a right and left bronchial artery.

1 Common bronchial trunk
2 Intercostal artery
3 Left bronchial branches
4 Reflux filling of left bronchial artery
5 Right bronchial artery
6 Tip of catheter in common bronchial arterial trunk
7 Tip of catheter in intercostobronchial trunk

(d) Azygos venogram.

In the thorax the vertebral veins drain into intercostal veins, while in the lumbar region the lumbar veins drain into the ascending lumbar veins. The right ascending lumbar vein becomes the azygos vein on entering the thorax, and the left ascending lumbar vein becomes the hemi-azygos vein. At the level of the fourth thoracic vertebra, the azygos vein turns anteriorly (the arch of the azygos) to enter the superior vena cava. The hemi-azygos vein crosses to join the azygos vein at the level of the eighth or ninth thoracic vertebral body. The accessory hemi-azygos vein is continuous with the hemi-azygos vein inferiorly and the left superior intercostal vein superiorly.

1 Accessory hemi-azygos vein
2 Azygos arch
3 Azygos vein
4 Hemi-azygos vein
5 Intercostal veins
6 Subtraction artefact caused by cardiac and catheter movement
7 Tip of catheter introduced via femoral vein into superior vena cava and azygos vein

5 Abdomen

Abdomen, supine projection.

1 Gas in caecum and ascending colon
2 Gas in descending colon
3 Gas in stomach
4 Left kidney
5 Left psoas muscle
6 Right kidney
7 Right psoas muscle
8 Twelfth rib

Abdomen, **(a)** demonstrating gas in stomach and first part of duodenum, **(b)** demonstrating a calcified lymph node, **(c)** demonstrating calcified pelvic veins (phleboliths), supine projections.

1 Antrum of stomach
2 Fundus
3 Greater curvature of stomach
4 Lesser curvature of stomach
5 Phlebolith
6 Rugae of stomach
7 Superior (first) part of duodenum (duodenal cap)
8 Calcified lymph mode

(a) Peroperative cholangiogram.

1	Catheter
2	Common bile duct
3	Common hepatic duct
4	Dorsal branch of right hepatic duct
5	Hepatopancreatic (Vater's) ampulla
6	Left hepatic duct
7	Pancreatic duct
8	Stump of cystic duct
9	Ventral branch of right hepatic duct

(b) Oral cholecystogram, with the patient prone, oblique image.

1	Body of gall bladder
2	Common bile duct
3	Common hepatic duct
4	Cystic duct
5	Fundus of gall bladder

(a)–(k) Abdomen, axial CT images.

1	Anterior segment of right lobe of liver	17	Hemi-azygos vein
2	Aorta	18	Hepatic artery
3	Azygos vein	19	Ileum
4	Body of pancreas	20	Inferior vena cava
5	Body of stomach	21	Jejunum
6	Coeliac trunk	22	Lateral segment of left lobe of liver
7	Common bile duct	23	Latissimus dorsi muscle
8	Descending (second) part of duodenum	24	Left colic (splenic) flexure
9	Descending colon	25	Left crus of diaphragm
10	Diaphragm	26	Left gastric artery
11	Erector spinae muscle	27	Left hepatic vein
12	Fissure for ligamentum venosum	28	Left kidney
13	Fundus of stomach	29	Left renal vein
14	Gall bladder	30	Left suprarenal gland
15	Greater curvature of stomach	31	Lesser curvature of stomach
16	Head of pancreas	32	Medial segment of left lobe of liver

33 Middle hepatic vein	**49** Right kidney
34 Neck of pancreas	**50** Right lobe of liver
35 Oesophagus	**51** Right renal artery
36 Pararenal fat	**52** Right renal vein
37 Perirenal fat	**53** Right suprarenal gland
38 Portal vein	**54** Serratus anterior muscle
39 Posterior segment of right lobe of liver	**55** Spleen
40 Psoas major muscle	**56** Splenic artery
41 Pyloric part of stomach	**57** Splenic vein
42 Quadratus lumborum muscle	**58** Superior (first) part of duodenum
43 Rectus abdominis muscle	**59** Superior mesenteric artery
44 Renal fascia	**60** Superior mesenteric vein
45 Renal pelvis	**61** Tail of pancreas
46 Right colic (hepatic) flexure	**62** Transverse colon
47 Right crus of diaphragm	**63** Trapezius muscle
48 Right hepatic vein	**64** Uncinate process of head of pancreas

(i)–(k) Abdomen, axial CT images.

1	Aorta	**15**	Left kidney
2	Ascending colon	**16**	Pararenal fat
3	Body of vertebra	**17**	Perirenal fat
4	Common iliac artery	**18**	Psoas major muscle
5	Descending colon	**19**	Quadratus lumborum
6	Erector spinae muscle		muscle
7	External oblique muscle	**20**	Rectus abdominis muscle
8	Gluteus medius muscle	**21**	Renal fascia
9	Horizontal (third) part of	**22**	Right crus of diaphragm
	duodenum	**23**	Right kidney
10	Ileum	**24**	Thecal sac
11	Ilium	**25**	Transversus abdominis
12	Inferior mesenteric artery		muscle
13	Inferior vena cava	**26**	Umbilicus
14	Internal oblique muscle	**27**	Ureter

(a)–(f) Abdomen, axial MR images.

1	Aorta	19	Left renal vein
2	Ascending colon	20	Pararenal fat
3	Body of vertebra	21	Perirenal fat
4	Descending colon	22	Posterior segment of right lobe
5	Erector spinae muscle		of liver
6	External oblique muscle	23	Psoas major muscle
7	Gonadal artery and vein	24	Quadratus lumborum muscle
8	Horizontal (third) part of	25	Rectus abdominis muscle
	duodenum	26	Renal fascia
9	Ileum	27	Right crus of diaphragm
10	Inferior mesenteric artery	28	Right kidney
11	Inferior mesenteric vein	29	Right renal artery
12	Inferior vena cava	30	Right renal vein
13	Internal oblique muscle	31	Superior mesenteric artery
14	Jejunum	32	Superior mesenteric vein
15	Latissimus dorsi muscle	33	Thecal sac
16	Left crus of diaphragm	34	Transversus abdominis muscle
17	Left kidney	35	Ureter
18	Left renal artery		

(d)–(f) Abdomen, axial MR images.

1	Ascending colon	**12**	Inferior mesenteric artery
2	Body of vertebra	**13**	Inferior mesenteric vein
3	Common iliac artery	**14**	Inferior vena cava
4	Common iliac vein	**15**	Internal oblique muscle
5	Descending colon	**16**	Intervertebral disc
6	Erector spinae muscle	**17**	Psoas major muscle
7	External oblique muscle	**18**	Quadratus lumborum muscle
8	Gluteus medius muscle	**19**	Rectus abdominis muscle
9	Gonadal artery and vein	**20**	Transversus abdominis muscle
10	Ileum		
11	Ilium	**21**	Ureter

(a)–(f) Abdomen, sagittal MR images.

1 Aorta	**18** Neck of pancreas
2 Body of pancreas	**19** Oesophagus
3 Body of stomach	**20** Perirenal fat
4 Body of vertebra	**21** Psoas major muscle
5 Coeliac trunk	**22** Quadratus lumborum
6 Common iliac artery	muscle
7 Diaphragm	**23** Rectus abdominis muscle
8 Erector spinae muscle	**24** Renal pelvis
9 Fundus of stomach	**25** Spleen
10 Horizontal (third) part of	**26** Splenic artery
duodenum	**27** Splenic vein
11 Ileum	**28** Superior mesenteric
12 Intervertebral disc	artery
13 Jejunum	**29** Tail of pancreas
14 Left kidney	**30** Tendinous intersection
15 Left renal artery	**31** Transverse colon
16 Left renal vein	**32** Ureter
17 Medial segment of left	**33** Xiphoid process of
lobe of liver	sternum

(d)–(f) Abdomen, sagittal MR images.

1	Anterior segment of right lobe of liver	**20**	Porta hepatis
2	Ascending colon	**21**	Portal vein
3	Caudate lobe of liver	**22**	Posterior segment of right lobe of liver
4	Common iliac artery	**23**	Psoas major muscle
5	Common iliac vein	**24**	Pyloric part of stomach
6	Descending (second) part of duodenum	**25**	Quadratus lumborum muscle
7	Diaphragm	**26**	Rectus abdominis muscle
8	Erector spinae muscle	**27**	Renal fascia
9	Gall bladder	**28**	Renal pelvis
10	Head of pancreas	**29**	Right colic (hepatic) flexure
11	Horizontal (third) part of duodenum	**30**	Right hepatic vein
12	Ileum	**31**	Right kidney
13	Ilium	**32**	Right renal artery
14	Inferior vena cava	**33**	Right renal vein
15	Lateral segment of left lobe of liver	**34**	Superior (first) part of duodenum
16	Left hepatic vein	**35**	Tendinous intersection
17	Middle hepatic vein	**36**	Transverse colon
18	Pararenal fat	**37**	Uncinate process of head of pancreas
19	Perirenal fat		

(a)–(f) Abdomen, coronal MR images.
• Note the small left renal cyst.

1 Aorta	**18** Psoas major muscle
2 Azygos vein	**19** Quadratus lumborum
3 Body of vertebra	muscle
4 External oblique muscle	**20** Renal cyst
5 Gluteus maximus muscle	**21** Renal fascia
6 Ilium	**22** Renal pelvis
7 Internal iliac artery	**23** Right crus of diaphragm
8 Internal oblique muscle	**24** Right kidney
9 Intervertebral disc	**25** Right lobe of liver
10 Lateral part (ala) of	**26** Right suprarenal gland
sacrum	**27** Sacro-iliac joint
11 Left atrium	**28** Spleen
12 Left crus of diaphragm	**29** Splenic artery
13 Left kidney	**30** Splenic vein
14 Left suprarenal gland	**31** Superior gluteal artery
15 Pararenal fat	**32** Thecal sac
16 Perirenal fat	**33** Transversus abdominis
17 Posterior segment of right	muscle
lobe of liver	**34** Ureter

(d)–(f) Abdomen, coronal MR images.

1	Anterior segment of right lobe of liver	**25**	Left crus of diaphragm
2	Aorta	**26**	Left kidney
3	Ascending colon	**27**	Left renal artery
4	Caudate lobe of liver	**28**	Left renal vein
5	Coeliac trunk	**29**	Left suprarenal gland
6	Common bile duct	**30**	Middle hepatic vein
7	Common iliac artery	**31**	Oesophagus
8	Common iliac vein	**32**	Porta hepatis
9	Descending (second) part of duodenum	**33**	Portal vein
10	Descending colon	**34**	Psoas major muscle
11	Diaphragm	**35**	Renal pelvis
12	External oblique muscle	**36**	Right atrium
13	Fundus of stomach	**37**	Right crus of diaphragm
14	Gall bladder	**38**	Right hepatic vein
15	Gastro-oesophageal junction	**39**	Right renal artery
16	Hepatic artery	**40**	Spleen
17	Ileocolic artery	**41**	Splenic artery
18	Iliotibial tract	**42**	Splenic vein
19	Ilium	**43**	Superior mesenteric artery
20	Inferior mesenteric artery	**44**	Tail of pancreas
21	Inferior mesenteric vein	**45**	Transverse colon
22	Inferior vena cava	**46**	Transversus abdominis muscle
23	Internal oblique muscle	**47**	Uncinate process of head of pancreas
24	Left atrium	**48**	Ureter

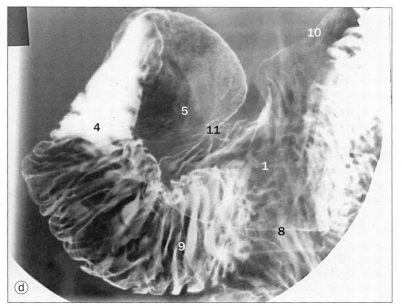

Abdomen. Double-contrast barium meals of stomach and duodenum, **(a)** and **(b)** with the patient supine (to show the mucosa of the stomach), **(c)** with the patient erect, **(d)** with the patient in a supine oblique position (to show the duodenum).

1	Antrum of stomach	**7**	Gas bubbles
2	Barium pooling in fundus of stomach	**8**	Greater curvature of stomach
3	Body of stomach	**9**	Horizontal (third) part of duodenum
4	Descending (second) part of duodenum	**10**	Lesser curvature of stomach
5	Duodenal cap (superior or first part of duodenum)	**11**	Region of pyloric canal
		12	Rugae of stomach
6	Fundus of stomach	**13**	Small bowel

Abdomen, barium follow-throughs, **(a)** with the patient supine, **(b)** showing a localised view of the terminal ileum, anteroposterior radiographs.

1 Caecum	**6** Right sacro-iliac joint
2 Compression device	**7** Stomach
3 Descending (second) part of duodenum	**8** Terminal ileum
4 Proximal ileum	**9** Valvulae conniventes (plicae circulares) of
5 Proximal jejunum	jejunum

Abdomen, double-contrast barium enema of the large bowel (colon).

1 Ascending portion of colon	**6** Right colic (hepatic) flexure of colon
2 Caecum	**7** Sacculations (haustrations) of colon
3 Descending portion of colon	**8** Sigmoid colon
4 Left colic (splenic) flexure of colon	**9** Terminal ileum
5 Rectum	**10** Transverse portion of colon

Abdominal ultrasound, (a)–(h) sagittal and parasagittal views, (i)–(l) transverse and transverse oblique views.

1	Abdominal aorta	6	Common bile duct
2	Body of pancreas	7	Cystic duct
3	Branch of hepatic vein	8	Fat in renal sinus
4	Branch of portal vein	9	Fundus of gall bladder
5	Coeliac trunk	10	Gall bladder

11	Head of pancreas
12	Hepatic artery
13	Hepatorenal recess
14	Inferior vena cava
15	Left dome of diaphragm

16	Left hepatic vein	23	Right dome of diaphragm	30	Spleen
17	Left lobe of liver	24	Right hepatic artery	31	Splenic vein
18	Left renal vein	25	Right hepatic vein	32	Superior mesenteric artery
19	Middle hepatic vein	26	Right kidney	33	Superior mesenteric vein
20	Neck of pancreas	27	Right lobe of liver	34	Tail of pancreas
21	Portal vein	28	Right renal artery	35	Vertebral body
22	Renal papilla	29	Right renal vein		

(a) and (b) Subtracted coeliac trunk arteriograms.

1 Dorsal pancreatic artery
2 Gastroduodenal artery
3 Hepatic artery
4 Left gastric artery
5 Left gastro-epiploic artery
6 Left hepatic artery
7 Pancreatica magna artery
8 Phrenic artery
9 Right gastro-epiploic artery
10 Right hepatic artery
11 Splenic artery
12 Superior pancreatico duodenal artery
13 Tip of catheter in coeliac trunk
14 Transverse pancreatic artery

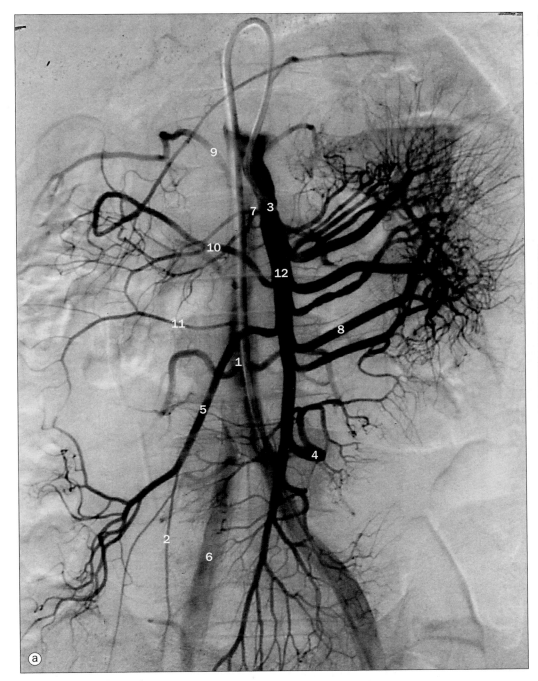

(a) Subtracted superior mesenteric arteriogram.

1 Aorta
2 Appendicular artery
3 Catheter with tip selectively in superior mesenteric artery
4 Ileal branches of superior mesenteric artery
5 Ileocolic artery
6 Iliac artery
7 Inferior pancreaticoduodenal artery
8 Jejunal branches of superior mesenteric artery
9 Lumbar arteries arising from abdominal aorta
10 Middle colic artery
11 Right colic artery
12 Superior mesenteric artery

(b) Gastric arteries, (c) gastric veins.

1 Catheter in origin of left gastric artery
2 Left gastric artery
3 Left gastric vein
4 Oesophageal branch of left gastric artery
5 Oesophageal branches of left gastric vein
6 Right gastric artery
7 Short gastric veins
8 Splenic vein

(a) Subtracted inferior mesenteric arteriogram.

(b) Venous phase of subtracted inferior mesenteric arteriogram.

(c) Inferior mesenteric arteriogram.

1	Ascending branch of left colic artery
2	Descending branch of left colic artery
3	Inferior mesenteric artery
4	Inferior mesenteric vein
5	Left colic artery
6	Left colic vein
7	Marginal artery of Drummond
8	Sigmoid arteries
9	Sigmoid vein
10	Superior rectal artery
11	Superior rectal vein
12	Tip of catheter in inferior mesenteric artery

(a) Indirect splenoportogram.

(b) and (c) Venous phase of superior mesenteric arteriogram.

1	Entry of superior mesenteric vein
2	Ileocolic vein
3	Jejunal vein
4	Left branch of portal vein
5	Portal vein
6	Right branch of portal vein
7	Site of entry of splenic vein
8	Spleen
9	Splenic vein
10	Superior mesenteric vein
11	Tip of catheter in splenic artery
12	Tip of catheter in superior mesenteric artery

(a) Subtracted hepatic arteriogram.

1	Anterior branch of superior pancreaticoduodenal artery
2	Dorsal pancreatic artery
3	Epiploic arteries
4	Gastroduodenal artery
5	Left branch of hepatic artery
6	Posterior branch of superior pancreaticoduodenal artery
7	Right branch of hepatic artery
8	Right gastro-epiploic artery
9	Superior pancreaticoduodenal artery
10	Tip of catheter in hepatic artery
11	Transverse pancreatic artery

(b) Subtracted hepatic venogram.

1	Inferior vena cava
2	Middle hepatic vein
3	Parenchyma of liver
4	Right hepatic vein
5	Tip of catheter in hepatic vein

(a) Endoscopic retrograde cholangiopancreatogram (ERCP).

1 Accessory pancreatic (Santorini's) duct
2 Ampullary part of pancreatic duct
3 Contrast and gas in descending (second) part of duodenum
4 Intralobular ducts
5 Main pancreatic duct

(b) Subtracted pancreatic arteriogram.

1 Anterior branch of inferior pancreatico duodenal artery
2 Anterior branch of superior pancreatico duodenal artery
3 Gastroduodenal artery
4 Left gastro-epiploic artery
5 Posterior branch of inferior pancreatico duodenal artery
6 Posterior branch of superior pancreatico duodenal artery
7 Right gastro-epiploic artery
8 Superior mesenteric artery
9 Tip of catheter in dorsal pancreatic artery
10 Transverse pancreatic artery

(a) Nephrographic phase of an excretion urogram.

1	Gas in stomach
2	Gas in transverse colon
3	Lateral border of right kidney
4	Lateral margin of left kidney
5	Left psoas muscle
6	Lower pole of left kidney
7	Lower pole of right kidney
8	Right psoas muscle
9	Upper pole of left kidney
10	Upper pole of right kidney

(b) Pyelographic phase of an excretion urogram.

1	Left ureter
2	Lower pole of left kidney
3	Major calyx
4	Minor calyx
5	Renal papilla
6	Renal pelvis
7	Upper pole of left kidney

(a) Renal arteriogram.

1 Arcuate arteries
2 Interlobar arteries
3 Lobar arteries
4 Main renal artery
5 Tip of catheter in renal artery

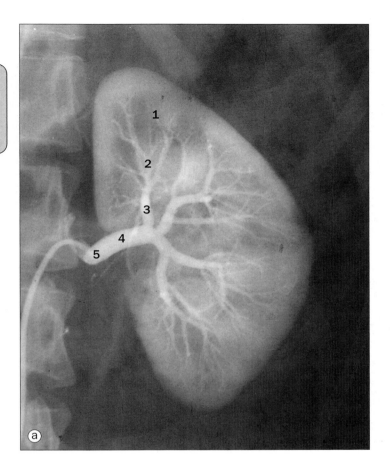

(b) Left renal venogram.

1 Arcuate veins
2 Catheter in left renal artery
3 Catheter in left renal vein
4 Inferior vena cava
5 Interlobar veins
6 Lobar veins
7 Main renal vein

(a) Left suprarenal arteriogram.

(b) Left suprarenal venogram.

Angiography of the suprarenal glands has been superseded by other imaging techniques. Although there is a wide variation, the arterial supply to the suprarenal glands is from three main arteries: the inferior suprarenal artery, which comes off the renal artery; the middle suprarenal artery, directly off the aorta; and the superior suprarenal artery, arising from the inferior phrenic artery.
Suprarenal venous sampling is still performed in some centres as part of the localisation of hormone-secreting tumours.

1 Catheter in origin of inferior phrenic artery	
2 Diaphragm	
3 Inferior phrenic artery	
4 Left suprarenal gland	
5 Superior suprarenal arteries	
6 Tip of nasogastric tube	

1 Adenoma in suprarenal gland	5 Left renal vein
2 Capsular veins	6 Left suprarenal vein
3 Diaphragm	7 Tip of catheter in left suprarenal vein
4 Inferior phrenic vein	8 Upper pole calyx

(c) and **(d)** Suprarenal glands, axial MR images.

1 Aorta	8 Inferior vena cava	15 Medial segment of left lobe of liver
2 Body of left suprarenal gland	9 Lateral limb of left suprarenal gland	16 Portal vein
3 Body of right suprarenal gland	10 Lateral limb of right suprarenal gland	17 Right crus of diaphragm
4 Body of vertebra	11 Left crus of diaphragm	18 Right kidney
5 Caudate lobe of liver	12 Left kidney	19 Right lobe of liver
6 Common bile duct	13 Medial limb of left suprarenal gland	20 Splenic artery
7 Hepatic artery	14 Medial limb of right suprarenal gland	21 Splenic vein

Abdominal aortogram.

 1 Abdominal aorta
 2 Accessory renal arteries
 3 Coeliac trunk
 4 Common iliac arteries
 5 Hepatic artery
 6 Ileocolic artery
 7 Jejunal branches of superior mesenteric artery
 8 Left gastric artery
 9 Left renal artery
10 Lumbar arteries
11 Right renal artery
12 Splenic artery
13 Superior mesenteric artery
14 Tip of pigtail catheter in abdominal aorta

Inferior vena cavogram.

1 Ascending lumbar vein
2 Common iliac vein
3 Entrance of hepatic veins
4 Entrance of renal veins
5 External iliac vein
6 Iliolumbar vein
7 Inferior vena cava
8 Internal iliac vein

Lymphangiograms, (a) of the thorax and upper abdomen, (b) of the paralumbar region.

1 Ascending lumbar chains
2 Cisterna chyli
3 Efferent inguinal lymphatics
4 External iliac nodes (early filling)
5 Inguinal nodes (early filling)
6 Terminal ampulla
7 Thoracic duct

Lymphangiogram of the pelvic region.
For key, see page 143.

6 Pelvis

(a) Pelvis and hips of an adult female, anteroposterior projection.
(b) and (c) Pelvis of a 17-year-old male, anteroposterior projections.

1 Anterior inferior iliac spine	7 Iliac crest	13 Pubic symphysis
2 Anterior sacral foramen	8 Ilium	14 Sacral crest
3 Anterior superior iliac spine	9 Inferior ramus of pubis	15 Sacro-iliac joint
4 Body of pubis	10 Ischial ramus	16 Segment of coccyx
5 Centre for iliac crest	11 Ischial spine	17 Superior ramus of pubis
6 Centre for ischial tuberosity	12 Obturator foramen	18 Tubercle of pubis

(a)–(h) Male pelvis, axial CT images.

1 Aorta	**11** External iliac vein
2 Ascending colon	**12** External oblique muscle
3 Bladder	**13** Gluteus maximus muscle
4 Caecum	**14** Gluteus medius muscle
5 Common iliac artery	**15** Gluteus minimus muscle
6 Common iliac vein	**16** Gonadal artery and vein
7 Descending colon	**17** Ileal loop
8 Dome of bladder	**18** Iliacus muscle
9 Dorsal sacral foramen	**19** Iliopsoas muscle
10 External iliac artery	**20** Ilium

21	Inferior mesenteric artery	32	Sacrum
22	Inferior vena cava	33	Sartorius muscle
23	Internal iliac artery	34	Sigmoid colon
24	Internal iliac vein	35	Superior gluteal artery and vein
25	Internal oblique muscle	36	Tensor fasciae latae muscle
26	Mesenteric fat	37	Terminal ileum
27	Piriformis muscle	38	Thecal sac
28	Psoas muscle	39	Transversus abdominis muscle
29	Rectus abdominis muscle	40	Umbilicus
30	Sacral plexus	41	Ureter
31	Sacro-iliac joint	42	Ventral sacral foramen

(a)–(i) Male pelvis, axial CT images.

1	Acetabular roof	23	Gluteus minimus muscle	45	Profunda femoris artery
2	Acetabulum	24	Gracilis muscle	46	Prostate
3	Adductor brevis muscle	25	Greater trochanter of femur	47	Pubic symphysis
4	Adductor longus muscle	26	Head of femur	48	Quadratus femoris muscle
5	Adductor magnus muscle	27	Iliopsoas muscle	49	Rectum
6	Anal canal	28	Iliotibial tract	50	Rectus abdominis muscle
7	Biceps femoris muscle	29	Inferior gluteal artery and vein	51	Rectus femoris muscle
8	Bladder	30	Inferior ramus of pubis	52	Sacrospinous ligament
9	Body of pubis	31	Internal pudendal artery and vein	53	Sacrum
10	Bulb of penis	32	Ischial spine	54	Sartorius muscle
11	Coccyx	33	Ischio-anal fossa	55	Sciatic nerve
12	Corpus cavernosum	34	Ischium	56	Semimembranosus muscle
13	Crus of corpus cavernosum	35	Lesser trochanter of femur	57	Seminal vesicle
14	Epididymis	36	Levator ani muscle	58	Semitendinosus muscle
15	External anal sphincter	37	Ligament of head of femur	59	Sigmoid colon
16	External iliac artery	38	Membranous urethra	60	Spermatic cord
17	External iliac vein	39	Neck of femur	61	Superficial femoral artery
18	Femoral artery	40	Obturator artery and vein	62	Superior ramus of pubis
19	Femoral vein	41	Obturator externus muscle	63	Tensor fasciae latae muscle
20	Gemellus muscle	42	Obturator internus muscle	64	Testis
21	Gluteus maximus muscle	43	Pectineus muscle	65	Vastus intermedius muscle
22	Gluteus medius muscle	44	Piriformis muscle	66	Vastus lateralis muscle

(a)–(f) Male pelvis, sagittal MR images.

1 Acetabulum	**16** Ejaculatory duct
2 Adductor brevis muscle	**17** Epididymis
3 Adductor longus muscle	**18** External iliac artery
4 Adductor magnus muscle	**19** External iliac vein
5 Anal canal	**20** Femoral artery
6 Aorta	**21** Fifth lumbar vertebra
7 Bladder	**22** First sacral segment
8 Bladder neck	**23** Gemellus muscle
9 Body of pubis	**24** Gluteus maximus muscle
10 Bulb of penis	**25** Gracilis muscle
11 Coccyx	**26** Iliacus muscle
12 Common iliac vein	**27** Iliopsoas muscle
13 Corpus cavernosum	**28** Ilium
14 Corpus spongiosum	**29** Inferior gluteal artery and vein
15 Descending colon	**30** Internal iliac artery

31 Internal iliac vein	**47** Quadratus lumborum muscle
32 Ischial spine	**48** Rectum
33 Ischial tuberosity	**49** Rectus abdominis muscle
34 Ischio-anal fossa	**50** Sacrospinous ligament
35 Ischium	**51** Sartorius muscle
36 Levator ani muscle	**52** Sciatic nerve
37 Lumbosacral disc	**53** Semimembranosus muscle
38 Median sacral artery	**54** Seminal vesicle
39 Membranous urethra	**55** Semitendinosus muscle
40 Obturator internus muscle	**56** Sigmoid colon
41 Pectineus muscle	**57** Spermatic cord
42 Penile urethra	**58** Superior gluteal artery and vein
43 Piriformis muscle	**59** Superior ramus of pubis
44 Prostate	**60** Testis
45 Prostatic urethra	**61** Thecal sac
46 Psoas muscle	

(a)–(h) Male pelvis, coronal MR images.

1 Acetabular roof	**15** External iliac artery
2 Acetabulum	**16** External iliac vein
3 Anal canal	**17** Fifth lumbar vertebra
4 Bladder	**18** Gemellus muscle
5 Branches of superior mesenteric artery	**19** Gluteus maximus muscle
6 Bulb of penis	**20** Gluteus medius muscle
7 Caecum	**21** Head of femur
8 Common iliac artery	**22** Iliacus muscle
9 Common iliac vein	**23** Iliopsoas muscle
10 Corpus cavernosum	**24** Ilium
11 Corpus spongiosum	**25** Inferior gluteal artery and vein
12 Crus of corpus cavernosum	**26** Inferior ramus of pubis
13 Descending colon	**27** Inferior vena cava
14 Ductus deferens (vas deferens)	**28** Internal iliac artery

29 Internal iliac vein	**44** Pubic symphysis
30 Internal pudendal artery and vein	**45** Quadratus femoris muscle
31 Ischial tuberosity	**46** Rectum
32 Ischio-anal fossa	**47** Sacral plexus
33 Ischium	**48** Sacro-iliac joint
34 Lateral part (ala) of sacrum	**49** Sacrum
35 Levator ani muscle	**50** Sciatic nerve
36 Lumbosacral disc	**51** Seminal vesicle
37 Median sacral artery	**52** Sigmoid colon
38 Obturator externus muscle	**53** Superior gluteal artery and vein
39 Obturator internus muscle	**54** Superior ramus of pubis
40 Pectineus muscle	**55** Tensor fasciae latae muscle
41 Piriformis muscle	**56** Thecal sac
42 Prostate	**57** Ventral sacral foramen
43 Psoas muscle	

(a)–(c) Male pelvis, coronal MR images.

1 Bladder	**11** Pectineus muscle
2 Corpus cavernosum	**12** Profunda femoris artery
3 Corpus spongiosum	**13** Pubic symphysis
4 External iliac artery	**14** Rectus abdominis muscle
5 External iliac vein	**15** Sartorius muscle
6 Femoral artery	**16** Spermatic cord
7 Femoral vein	**17** Superficial epigastric artery
8 Ileal loop	**18** Superior ramus of pubis
9 Iliopsoas muscle	**19** Tendinous intersection
10 Mesenteric fat	**20** Testis

(a)–(d) Male pelvis, axial MR images.

1 Acetabulum	**14** Iliopsoas muscle	**27** Pectineus muscle
2 Anal canal	**15** Inferior gluteal artery and vein	**28** Piriformis muscle
3 Bladder	**16** Internal iliac artery	**29** Prostate
4 Body of pubis	**17** Internal iliac vein	**30** Pubic symphysis
5 Coccyx	**18** Internal pudendal artery and vein	**31** Rectum
6 External iliac artery	**19** Ischio-anal fossa	**32** Rectus abdominis muscle
7 External iliac vein	**20** Ischium	**33** Rectus femoris muscle
8 Femoral artery	**21** Levator ani muscle	**34** Sacrospinous ligament
9 Femoral nerve	**22** Ligament of head of femur	**35** Sartorius muscle
10 Femoral vein	**23** Neck of femur	**36** Sciatic nerve
11 Gluteus maximus muscle	**24** Obturator artery and vein	**37** Seminal vesicle
12 Greater trochanter of femur	**25** Obturator externus muscle	**38** Spermatic cord
13 Head of femur	**26** Obturator internus muscle	

(e)–(f) Male pelvis, axial MR images.

1 Adductor longus muscle	**13** Neck of femur
2 Anal canal	**14** Obturator externus muscle
3 Body of pubis	**15** Obturator internus muscle
4 Femoral artery	**16** Pectineus muscle
5 Femoral nerve	**17** Prostate
6 Femoral vein	**18** Pubic symphysis
7 Gluteus maximus muscle	**19** Quadratus femoris muscle
8 Iliopsoas muscle	**20** Rectus femoris muscle
9 Internal pudendal artery and vein	**21** Sartorius muscle
10 Ischio-anal fossa	**22** Sciatic nerve
11 Ischium	**23** Spermatic cord
12 Levator ani muscle	**24** Tensor fasciae latae muscle

(a)–(c) Female pelvis, axial MR images.

1	Acetabular roof	16	Ovary
2	Bladder	17	Piriformis muscle
3	Broad ligament	18	Posterior fornix of vagina
4	Cavity of uterus	19	Rectum
5	Coccyx	20	Rectus abdominis muscle
6	External iliac artery and vein	21	Round ligament
7	External os of cervix	22	Sacrospinous ligament
8	Fundus of uterus	23	Sacrum
9	Gluteus maximus muscle	24	Sigmoid colon
10	Head of femur	25	Uterine artery
11	Iliopsoas muscle	26	Uterine tube
12	Internal iliac artery and vein	27	Uterosacral ligament
13	Internal os of cervix	28	Vagina
14	Myometrium of uterus	29	Wall of cervix
15	Obturator internus muscle		

(d)–(f) Female pelvis, axial MR images.

1	Acetabulum	**16**	Levator ani muscle
2	Anal canal	**17**	Obturator externus muscle
3	Bladder	**18**	Obturator internus muscle
4	Body of pubis	**19**	Pectineus muscle
5	Coccyx	**20**	Profunda femoris artery
6	Femoral artery	**21**	Pubic symphysis
7	Femoral nerve	**22**	Quadratus femoris muscle
8	Femoral vein	**23**	Rectus abdominis muscle
9	Gluteus maximus muscle	**24**	Rectus femoris muscle
10	Head of femur	**25**	Sartorius muscle
11	Iliopsoas muscle	**26**	Sciatic nerve
12	Internal pudendal artery and vein	**27**	Superficial femoral artery
13	Ischial spine	**28**	Superficial femoral vein
14	Ischio-anal fossa	**29**	Tensor fasciae latae muscle
15	Ischium	**30**	Urethra
		31	Vagina

(a)–(c) Female pelvis, sagittal MR images.

1 Anterior fornix of vagina	16 Ischio-anal fossa
2 Bladder	17 Levator ani muscle
3 Body of pubis	18 Myometrium of uterus
4 Body of uterus	19 Obturator internus muscle
5 Cavity of uterus	20 Ovary
6 Coccyx	21 Piriformis muscle
7 Endocervical canal of cervix	22 Posterior fornix of vagina
8 Endometrium	23 Recto-uterine pouch
9 External iliac artery and vein	24 Rectus abdominis muscle
10 External os of cervix	25 Sacrum
11 Fundus of uterus	26 Sigmoid colon
12 Gluteus maximus muscle	27 Thecal sac
13 Ileum	28 Vagina
14 Internal iliac artery and vein	29 Vesico-uterine pouch
15 Internal os of cervix	30 Wall of cervix

(d)–(f) Female pelvis, sagittal MR images.

1	Anal canal	**15**	Ovary
2	Bladder	**16**	Psoas muscle
3	Body of pubis	**17**	Pubic symphysis
4	Cavity of uterus	**18**	Recto-uterine pouch
5	Coccyx	**19**	Rectum
6	Endometrium	**20**	Rectus abdominis muscle
7	Gluteus maximus muscle	**21**	Sacrum
8	Ileum	**22**	Sigmoid colon
9	Internal iliac artery and vein	**23**	Urethra
10	Ischio-anal fossa	**24**	Uterine tube
11	Labium majus	**25**	Vagina
12	Levator ani muscle	**26**	Vesico-uterine pouch
13	Myometrium of uterus	**27**	Wall of cervix
14	Obturator internus muscle		

1 Bladder	**14** Labium majus
2 Cavity of uterus	**15** Myometrium of uterus
3 Clitoris	**16** Obturator internus muscle
4 Common iliac artery	**17** Ovary
5 Common iliac vein	**18** Psoas muscle
6 Endometrium	**19** Pubic symphysis
7 Gluteus medius muscle	**20** Round ligament
8 Gluteus minimus muscle	**21** Sigmoid colon
9 Head of femur	**22** Superior ramus of pubis
10 Ileum	**23** Urethra
11 Iliacus muscle	**24** Urogenital diaphragm
12 Ilium	**25** Uterine tube
13 Labia minora	**26** Vagina

(a)–(c) Female pelvis, coronal MR images.

1	Anal canal	**12**	Obturator externus muscle
2	Cavity of uterus	**13**	Obturator internus muscle
3	Endometrium	**14**	Ovary
4	Greater trochanter of femur	**15**	Quadratus femoris muscle
5	Head of femur	**16**	Rectum
6	Ilium	**17**	Sacro-iliac joint
7	Inferior gemellus muscle	**18**	Sacrum
8	Ischio-anal fossa	**19**	Sigmoid colon
9	Lesser trochanter of femur	**20**	Superior gemellus muscle
10	Levator ani muscle	**21**	Vagina
11	Myometrium of uterus		

(d)–(f) Female pelvis, coronal MR images.

Subtracted pelvic arteriogram.

This anteroposterior film of the pelvis demonstrates both the internal and the external iliac arteries and their branches. Many of the vessels are superimposed: to see them more clearly oblique projections could be obtained. The contrast medium injected into the arteries is excreted by the kidneys, and a full bladder may obscure the branches. Selective catheterisation of the internal and external iliac arteries using a preshaped catheter gives better detail without superimposition of the vessels.

1 Anterior trunk of internal iliac artery	**10** Lateral circumflex femoral artery
2 Catheter introduced into distal abdominal aorta via right femoral artery	**11** Lateral sacral artery
	12 Median sacral artery
3 Common iliac artery	**13** Obturator artery
4 Deep circumflex iliac artery	**14** Position of uterus
5 External iliac artery	**15** Posterior trunk of internal iliac artery
6 Iliolumbar artery	**16** Profunda femoris artery
7 Inferior gluteal artery	**17** Superficial femoral artery
8 Inferior mesenteric artery	**18** Superior gluteal artery
9 Internal iliac artery	**19** Superior vesical artery
	20 Uterine artery

Female pelvic venogram.

1 Anterior division of internal iliac vein
2 Bladder containing contrast medium
3 Catheter introduced via right femoral vein, with tip in left internal iliac vein
4 Inferior gluteal veins
5 Obturator veins
6 Sacral plexus of veins
7 Sterilisation clips
8 Superior gluteal veins

(a) and (b) Right testicular venograms.

The gonadal veins drain into one or two main veins via a venous plexus. On the left, the main vein drains into the left renal vein. It may occasionally communicate with the inferior mesenteric vein and drain into the portal venous system. On the right, the main vein usually drains into the inferior vena cava directly (as in the case illustrated), but it can drain into the right renal vein.

1 Bladder
2 Common iliac veins
3 Inferior vena cava
4 Pampiniform plexus of veins
5 Pampiniform plexus of veins (undescended testis in inguinal canal)
6 Renal capsular veins
7 Right testicular vein
8 Tip of catheter in right testicular vein, introduced via left femoral vein
9 Ureter

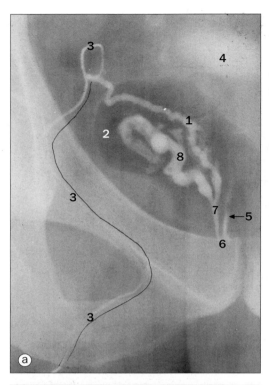

(a) Seminal vesiculogram.

1 Ampulla of ductus deferens
2 Colonic gas
3 Ductus deferens (vas deferens)
4 Full urinary bladder
5 Left ejaculatory duct
6 Position of seminal colliculus (verumontanum)
7 Right ejaculatory duct
8 Seminal vesicle

Rectal ultrasound of the prostate, (b) axial scan through bladder base, (c) axial scan through mid-prostate, (d) sagittal scan, right lobe laterally, (e) sagittal midline scan.

1 Ampulla of ductus deferens
2 Bladder
3 Course of urethra
4 Distal urethra
5 Ejaculatory duct
6 Left seminal vesicle
7 Peripheral zone of prostate
8 Rectal wall
9 Right seminal vesicle
10 Seminal vesicle
11 Transducer
12 Transitional zone of prostate

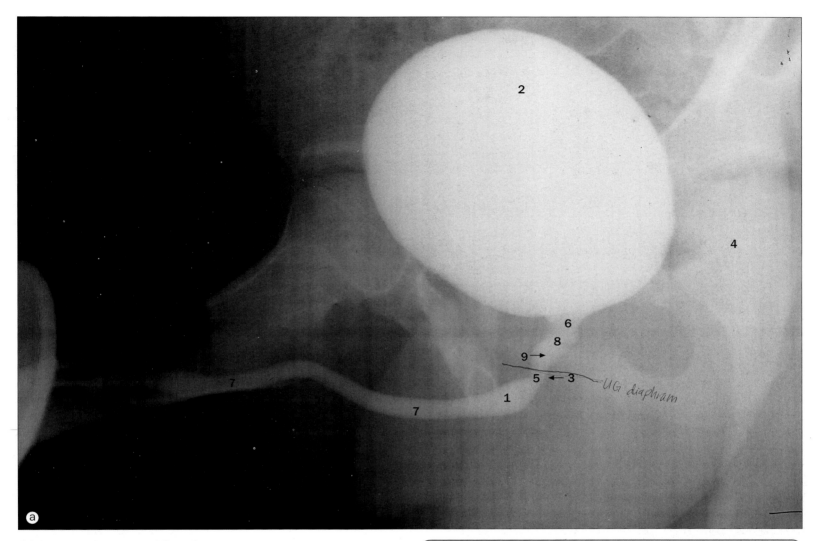

(a)

(a) Male urethrogram, oblique image.
(b) Penile arteriogram.
(c) Cavernosogram.

1	Bulbous urethra	6	Neck of urinary bladder
2	Contrast in urinary bladder	7	Penile urethra
3	External sphincter (sphincter urethrae)	8	Prostatic urethra
4	Head of femur	9	Seminal colliculus (verumontanum)
5	Membranous urethra		

(b)

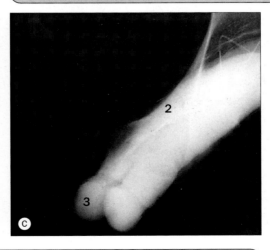

(c)

1	Artery of the penis	5	Dorsal artery of the penis
2	Corpus cavernosum	6	Internal pudendal artery
3	Crus of corpus cavernosum	7	Perineal artery
4	Deep artery of the penis		

(a)–(f) Testicular MR images.

1 Corpus cavernosum
2 Corpus spongiosum
3 Crus of corpus cavernosum
4 Dorsal artery of the penis
5 Ductus deferens (vas deferens)
6 Epididymis
7 Pampiniform plexus of veins
8 Penis
9 Scrotum
10 Spermatic cord
11 Testis
12 Tunica albuginea
13 Urethra

Hysterosalpingograms, (a) immediately after injection, (b) some minutes after injection.

1 Ampulla of uterine tube
2 Body of uterus
3 Cervix of uterus
4 Contrast spillage into peritoneal cavity
5 Cornu of uterus
6 Fundus of uterus
7 Isthmus of uterine tube
8 Speculum in vagina

(c) and (d) transvaginal ultrasound of the uterus.
(e) and (f) sagittal MR images, female pelvis.

1 Anal canal
2 Bladder
3 Cavity of uterus
4 Cervix of uterus
5 Coccyx
6 Endometrium
7 Fundus of uterus
8 Labium majus
9 Myometrium of uterus
10 Ovarian follicle
11 Ovary
12 Pubic symphysis
13 Recto-uterine pouch
14 Rectum
15 Round ligament of uterus
16 Sacrum
17 Sigmoid colon
18 Thecal sac
19 Urethra
20 Vagina
21 Vesico-uterine pouch
22 Wall of cervix

Fetal ultrasound, second trimester (a) cord insertion, (b) and (c) skull, (d) abdomen, (e) and (f) spine.

1	Abdominal aorta	**16**	Posterior elements of vertebrae
2	Abdominal circumference measurement	**17**	Ribs
3	Amniotic fluid	**18**	Skull
4	Anterior abdominal wall	**19**	Spinal canal
5	Biparietal diameter measurement	**20**	Spinal cord
6	Cavum septum pellucidum	**21**	Spine
7	Cerebellum	**22**	Stomach
8	Choroid plexus	**23**	Thalamus
9	Cisterna magna (cerebellomedullary cistern)	**24**	Thigh
10	Coronal suture	**25**	Umbilical cord
11	Falx cerebri	**26**	Umbilical vein
12	Femur	**27**	Umbilicus
13	Lambdoid suture	**28**	Uterine wall
14	Liver	**29**	Vertebral body
15	Placenta		

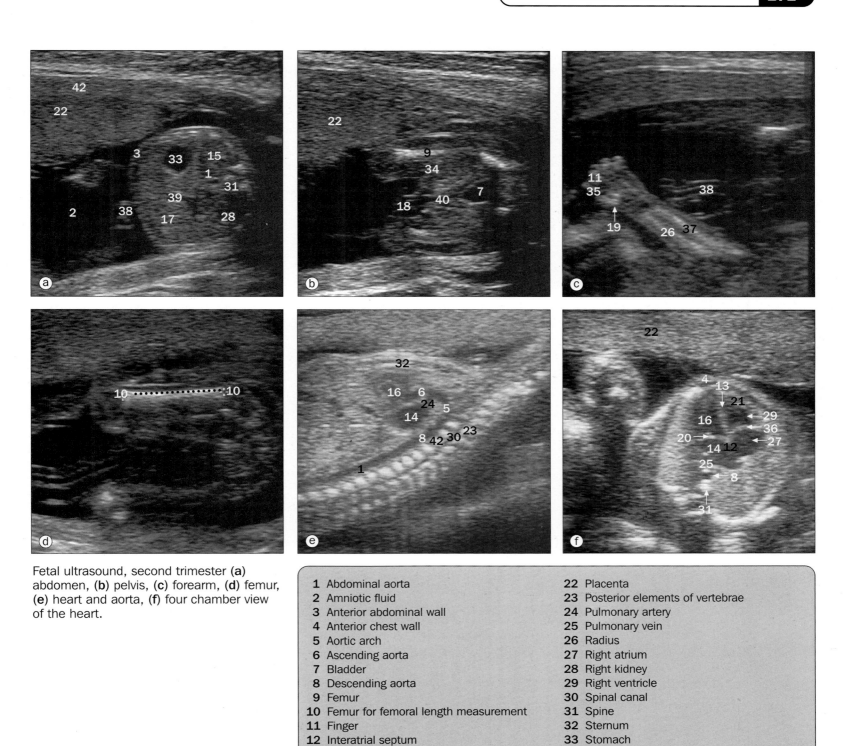

Fetal ultrasound, second trimester (a) abdomen, (b) pelvis, (c) forearm, (d) femur, (e) heart and aorta, (f) four chamber view of the heart.

1 Abdominal aorta	22 Placenta
2 Amniotic fluid	23 Posterior elements of vertebrae
3 Anterior abdominal wall	24 Pulmonary artery
4 Anterior chest wall	25 Pulmonary vein
5 Aortic arch	26 Radius
6 Ascending aorta	27 Right atrium
7 Bladder	28 Right kidney
8 Descending aorta	29 Right ventricle
9 Femur	30 Spinal canal
10 Femur for femoral length measurement	31 Spine
11 Finger	32 Sternum
12 Interatrial septum	33 Stomach
13 Interventricular septum	34 Thigh
14 Left atrium	35 Thumb
15 Left kidney	36 Tricuspid valve
16 Left ventricle	37 Ulna
17 Liver	38 Umbilical cord
18 Male external genitalia	39 Umbilical vein
19 Metacarpal shaft	40 Urethra
20 Mitral valve	41 Uterine wall
21 Moderator band	42 Vertebral body

7 Lower limb

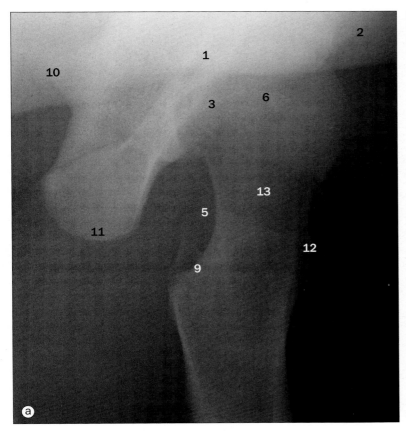

(a) Hip (for neck of femur), lateral projection.

(b) Hip, lateral projection.

(c) Hip, antero-posterior projection.

1	Acetabulum
2	Anterior inferior iliac spine
3	Epiphysial line
4	Fovea
5	Greater trochanter of femur
6	Head of femur
7	Inferior ramus of pubis
8	Intertrochanteric crest of femur
9	Intertrochanteric line
10	Ischial spine
11	Ischial tuberosity
12	Lesser trochanter of femur
13	Neck of femur
14	Obturator foramen
15	Pubic symphysis
16	Superior ramus of pubis

Pelvis, (a) of a 2-month-old boy, (b) of a 1-year-old boy, (c) of an 11-year-old boy, anteroposterior projections.

1	Centre for greater trochanter
2	Centre for head of femur (femoral capital epiphysis)
3	Centre for lesser trochanter
4	Epiphysial line
5	Femur
6	Ilium
7	Ischium
8	Neck of femur
9	Pubic symphysis
10	Pubis
11	Triradiate cartilage
12	Unossified junction between ischium and pubis

INNOMINATE (HIP)	Appears	Fused
Ilium	2–3 miu	7–9 yrs
Ischium	4 miu	7–9 yrs
Pubis	4 miu	7–9 yrs
Acetabulum	11–14 yrs	15–25 yrs
Ant. sup. iliac spine	Puberty	15–25 yrs
Iliac crest/sup. spines	Puberty	15–25 yrs
Ischial tuberosity	Puberty +	15–25 yrs
FEMUR (c)		
Shaft	7 wiu	
Head	4–6 mths	14–18 yrs
Greater trochanter	2–4 yrs	14–18 yrs
Lesser trochanter	10–12 yrs	14–18 yrs
Distal end	9 miu	17–19 yrs

Knee, (a) anteroposterior projection, (b) lateral projection,
(c) Patella, inferosuperior (skyline) projection.

1	Apex (styloid process) of fibula
2	Epiphysial line
3	Fabella
4	Femur
5	Head of fibula
6	Intercondylar fossa
7	Lateral condyle of femur
8	Lateral condyle of tibia
9	Lateral epicondyle of femur
10	Medial condyle of femur
11	Medial condyle of tibia
12	Medial epicondyle of femur
13	Patella
14	Tibia
15	Tubercles of intercondylar eminence
16	Tuberosity of tibia

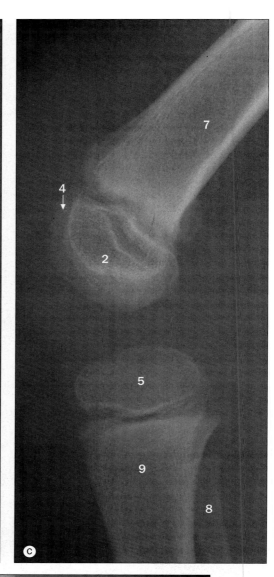

Knee, **(a)** of a 1-year-old boy, **(b)** and **(c)** of a 6-year-old boy, **(d)** and **(e)** of a 12-year-old boy.

PATELLA (c)	Appears	Fused
1–3 centres	3–5 yrs	Puberty
TIBIA (c)		
Shaft	7 wiu	
Proximal/plateau	9 miu	16–18 yrs
Tuberosity	10–12 yrs	12–14 yrs
Distal end	4 mths–1 yr	15–17 yrs
FIBULA (c)		
Shaft	8 wiu	
Proximal end/head	2–4 yrs	17–19 yrs
Distal end	6 mths–1 yr	15–17 yrs

1	Antero-inferior extension of proximal tibial centre for tuberosity of tibia	**5**	Centre for proximal tibia
2	Centre for distal femur	**6**	Epiphysial line
3	Centre for head of fibula	**7**	Femur
4	Centre for patella	**8**	Fibula
		9	Tibia

Ankle, (a) anteroposterior projection, (b) lateral projection. (c) Calcaneus, axial projection.

1	Calcaneus	**10**	Medial malleolus of tibia
2	Cuboid	**11**	Medial process of calcaneus
3	Fibula	**12**	Medial tubercle of talus
4	Head of talus	**13**	Navicular
5	Lateral cuneiform	**14**	Region of inferior tibiofibular joint
6	Lateral malleolus of fibula	**15**	Sustentaculum tali of calcaneus
7	Lateral process of calcaneus	**16**	Talus
8	Lateral tubercle of talus	**17**	Tibia
9	Medial malleolus	**18**	Tuberosity of base of fifth metatarsal

Ankle, (a) and (b) of a 3-year-old boy, (c) and (d) of a 5-year-old boy, (e) and (f) of a 13-year-old boy.

TARSAL BONES (c)	Appears	Fused
Calcaneus	3 miu	14–16 yrs
Talus	6 miu	
Navicular	3 yrs	
Cuneiform lateral	6 mths–1 yr	
Cuneiform intermediate	2–3 yrs	
Cuneiform medial	1–2 yrs	
Cuboid	9 miu	

1	Calcaneus	**7**	Fibula
2	Centre for distal fibula	**8**	Intermediate cuneiform
3	Centre for distal tibia	**9**	Lateral cuneiform
4	Centre for posterior aspect of calcaneus	**10**	Navicular
5	Cuboid	**11**	Talus
6	Epiphysial line	**12**	Tibia

1 Calcaneus
2 Cuboid
3 Distal phalanx of second toe
4 First metatarsal
5 Intermediate cuneiform
6 Lateral cuneiform
7 Medial cuneiform
8 Middle phalanx of second toe
9 Navicular
10 Proximal phalanx of second toe
11 Sesamoid bones in flexor hallucis brevis muscle
12 Talus
13 Tuberosity of base of fifth metatarsal

Foot, (a) dorsoplantar projection, (b) dorsoplantar oblique projection.

Foot, **(a)** of a 1-year-old boy, **(b)** of a 3-year-old boy, **(c)** of a 5-year-old boy, **(d)** of a 14-year-old boy.

1 Calcaneus
2 Centre for distal fibula
3 Centre for distal phalanx of second toe
4 Centre for distal tibia
5 Centre for first metatarsal
6 Centre for middle phalanx of second toe
7 Centre for posterior aspect of calcaneus
8 Centre for proximal phalanx of second toe
9 Centre for second metatarsal (applies to second to fifth metatarsal)
10 Centre for tuberosity of base of fifth metatarsal
11 Cuboid
12 Intermediate cuneiform
13 Lateral cuneiform
14 Medial cuneiform
15 Navicular
16 Talus

METATARSALS (c)	Appears	Fused
Shafts	9 wiu	
Heads (2–5) or base (1)	3–4 yrs	17–20 yrs
Tuberosity of 5	10–12 yrs	13–15 yrs
PHALANGES (c)		
Shaft	9–12 wiu	
Bases (variable)	1–6 yrs	14–18 yrs

(a) Femoral arteriogram.

The femoropopliteal and tibial arteries are imaged by catheterising the distal abdominal aorta and injecting contrast medium. The column of contrast is then followed as it passes down the legs. If only one leg is to be imaged, an injection into the ipsilateral femoral artery suffices. The external iliac artery continues as the common femoral artery, which originates deep to the inguinal ligament, dividing into the superficial and deep (profunda) femoral arteries. An oblique view is often useful to image the femoral bifurcation and to identify atheroma at the origins of these vessels.

1 Catheter introduced into distal abdominal aorta via left femoral artery
2 Common femoral artery
3 Lateral circumflex femoral artery
4 Medial circumflex femoral artery
5 Perforating artery
6 Profunda femoris artery
7 Superficial femoral artery

(b) Popliteal arteriogram.

The superficial femoral artery becomes the popliteal artery as it passes through the hiatus in the adductor magnus muscle. The popliteal artery terminates at the lower border of the popliteus muscle, dividing into the anterior and posterior tibial arteries.

1 Anterior tibial artery
2 Inferior lateral genicular artery
3 Inferior medial genicular artery
4 Muscular branches of anterior tibial artery
5 Muscular branches of posterior tibial artery
6 Peroneal artery
7 Popliteal artery
8 Posterior tibial artery
9 Superior lateral genicular artery
10 Superior medial genicular artery

(a) Popliteal arteriogram. (b) Foot arteriogram, lateral image.
(c) Foot venogram.

1 Anterior tibial artery
2 Dorsal venous arch
3 Dorsalis pedis artery
4 Great saphenous vein
5 Inferior lateral genicular artery
6 Inferior medial genicular artery
7 Lateral marginal vein
8 Lateral plantar artery
9 Medial calcaneal artery
10 Medial marginal vein
11 Medial plantar artery
12 Muscular branches of anterior tibial artery
13 Muscular branches of posterior tibial artery
14 Peroneal artery
15 Plantar arch
16 Plantar cutaneous venous plexus
17 Popliteal artery
18 Posterior tibial artery
19 Posterior tibial artery
20 Small saphenous vein
21 Superior medial genicular artery

(a)–(c) Lower limb venograms.

1 Anterior tibial vein
2 Femoral vein
3 Great (long) saphenous vein
4 Lateral circumflex vein
5 Muscular tributary of femoral vein
6 Perforating vein
7 Popliteal vein
8 Posterior tibial veins
9 Venous valves

(a)–(f) Thigh, axial MR images.

1 Adductor brevis muscle	**12** Femoral vein
2 Adductor longus muscle	**13** Femur
3 Adductor magnus muscle	**14** Gluteus maximus muscle
4 Anal canal	**15** Gracilis muscle
5 Articular muscle of the knee	**16** Great (long) saphenous vein
6 Biceps femoris muscle	**17** Iliopsoas muscle
7 Common peroneal nerve	**18** Iliotibial tract
8 Corpus cavernosum	**19** Inferior ramus of pubis
9 Crus of corpus cavernosum	**20** Ischial tuberosity
10 Femoral artery	**21** Ischio-anal fossa
11 Femoral nerve	**22** Lateral intermuscular septum

23	Levator ani muscle	**34**	Sciatic nerve
24	Long head of biceps femoris muscle	**35**	Semimembranosus muscle
25	Obturator externus muscle	**36**	Semitendinosus muscle
26	Obturator internus muscle	**37**	Short head of biceps femoris muscle
27	Pectineus muscle	**38**	Spermatic cord
28	Popliteal artery	**39**	Tendon of quadriceps muscle
29	Popliteal vein	**40**	Tensor fasciae latae muscle
30	Profunda femoris artery	**41**	Tibial nerve
31	Prostate	**42**	Vastus intermedius muscle
32	Rectus femoris muscle	**43**	Vastus lateralis muscle
33	Sartorius muscle	**44**	Vastus medialis muscle

(a)–(f) Thigh, sagittal MR images.

1 Acetabulum	14 Popliteal artery
2 Adductor longus muscle	15 Popliteal vein
3 Adductor magnus muscle	16 Quadratus femoris muscle
4 Biceps femoris muscle	17 Rectus femoris muscle
5 Femoral artery	18 Sartorius muscle
6 Femur	19 Semimembranosus muscle
7 Gluteus maximus muscle	20 Semitendinosus muscle
8 Head of femur	21 Subsartorial canal (Hunter's canal)
9 Iliopsoas muscle	22 Tendon of quadriceps muscle
10 Lateral head of gastrocnemius muscle	23 Vastus intermedius muscle
11 Obturator externus muscle	24 Vastus lateralis muscle
12 Pectineus muscle	25 Vastus medialis muscle
13 Piriformis muscle	

(a)–(f)) Thigh, coronal MR images.

1 Adductor brevis muscle	**18** Ischio-anal fossa
2 Adductor longus muscle	**19** Ischium
3 Adductor magnus muscle	**20** Lateral intermuscular septum
4 Anal canal	**21** Levator ani muscle
5 Biceps femoris muscle	**22** Neck of femur
6 Femoral artery	**23** Obturator externus muscle
7 Femur	**24** Obturator internus muscle
8 Gemellus muscle	**25** Pectineus muscle
9 Gluteus maximus muscle	**26** Profunda femoris artery
10 Gluteus medius muscle	**27** Quadratus femoris muscle
11 Gluteus minimus muscle	**28** Rectum
12 Gracilis muscle	**29** Rectus femoris muscle
13 Greater trochanter of femur	**30** Sartorius muscle
14 Head of femur	**31** Semimembranosus muscle
15 Iliopsoas muscle	**32** Semitendinosus muscle
16 Iliotibial tract	**33** Vastus intermedius muscle
17 Ischial tuberosity	**34** Vastus lateralis muscle

(a)–(e) Knee, axial MR images.

1	Anterior cruciate ligament	21	Patella
2	Biceps femoris muscle	22	Patellar tendon
3	Common peroneal nerve	23	Plantaris muscle
4	Deep fascia of the leg	24	Popliteal artery
5	Femur	25	Popliteal vein
6	Gracilis muscle	26	Popliteus muscle
7	Great saphenous vein	27	Posterior cruciate ligament
8	Head of fibula	28	Sartorius muscle
9	Iliotibial tract	29	Semimembranosus muscle
10	Infrapatellar fat pad	30	Short saphenous vein
11	Lateral collateral ligament	31	Tendon gracilis muscle
12	Lateral condyle of femur	32	Tendon of gracilis muscle
13	Lateral head of gastrocnemius muscle	33	Tendon of sartorius muscle
14	Lateral patellar retinaculum	34	Tendon of semimembranosus muscle
15	Lateral tibial plateau	35	Tendon of semitendinosus muscle
16	Medial collateral ligament	36	Tibia
17	Medial condyle of femur	37	Tibial nerve
18	Medial head of gastrocnemius muscle	38	Tibial tubercle
19	Medial patellar retinaculum	39	Vastus lateralis muscle
20	Medial tibial plateau	40	Vastus medialis muscle

(a)–(c) Knee, sagittal MR images.

1	Anterior cruciate ligament
2	Anterior horn of lateral meniscus
3	Femur
4	Head of fibula
5	Infrapatellar fat pad
6	Intercondylar notch
7	Lateral condyle of femur
8	Lateral condyle of tibia
9	Lateral head of gastrocnemius muscle
10	Patella
11	Patellar tendon
12	Plantaris muscle
13	Popliteal artery and vein
14	Popliteus muscle
15	Posterior cruciate ligament
16	Posterior horn of lateral meniscus
17	Posterior meniscofemoral ligament
18	Short head of biceps femoris muscle
19	Soleus muscle
20	Superior lateral genicular artery
21	Tendon of popliteus muscle
22	Tendon of quadriceps muscle
23	Tibia
24	Tibial tubercle
25	Tibialis anterior muscle
26	Tibiofibular joint
27	Vastus lateralis muscle

(d)–(f) Knee, sagittal MR images.

1	Anterior horn of medial meniscus
2	Articular cartilage
3	Femur
4	Inferior medial genicular artery
5	Medial condyle of femur
6	Medial condyle of tibia
7	Medial head of gastrocnemius muscle
8	Patella
9	Popliteus muscle
10	Posterior cruciate ligament
11	Posterior horn of medial meniscus
12	Semimembranosus muscle
13	Soleus muscle
14	Superior medial genicular artery
15	Tendon of popliteus muscle
16	Tendon of semitendinosus muscle
17	Tibia
18	Vastus medialis muscle

(a)–(f) Knee, coronal MR images.

1 Anterior cruciate ligament
2 Anterior horn of lateral meniscus
3 Anterior horn of medial meniscus
4 Biceps femoris muscle
5 Great (long) saphenous vein
6 Head of fibula
7 Iliotibial tract
8 Inferior medial genicular artery
9 Intercondylar notch
10 Lateral collateral ligament
11 Lateral condyle of femur
12 Lateral condyle of tibia
13 Lateral meniscus
14 Medial collateral ligament
15 Medial condyle of femur
16 Medial condyle of tibia
17 Medial head of gastrocnemius muscle
18 Medial meniscus
19 Posterior cruciate ligament
20 Sartorius muscle
21 Superior lateral genicular artery
22 Tibialis anterior muscle
23 Tibiofibular joint
24 Vastus lateralis muscle
25 Vastus medialis muscle

(d)–(f) Knee, coronal MR images.

1 Biceps femoris muscle
2 Common peroneal nerve
3 Gracilis muscle
4 Great (long) saphenous vein
5 Head of fibula
6 Lateral condyle of femur
7 Lateral condyle of tibia
8 Lateral head of gastrocnemius muscle
9 Medial condyle of femur
10 Medial condyle of tibia
11 Medial head of gastrocnemius muscle
12 Popliteal artery and vein
13 Popliteus muscle
14 Posterior horn of lateral meniscus
15 Posterior horn of medial meniscus
16 Posterior meniscofemoral ligament
17 Sartorius muscle
18 Semimembranosus muscle
19 Soleus muscle
20 Tendon of gracilis muscle
21 Tendon of semitendinosus muscle
22 Tibial nerve
23 Tibiofibular joint

(a)–(e) Calf, axial MR images.

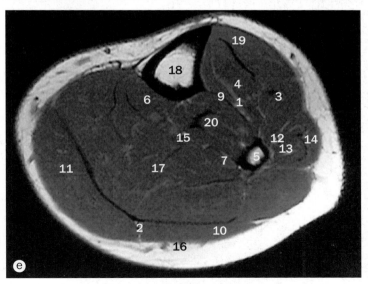

1 Anterior tibial artery	**10** Lateral head of gastrocnemius muscle
2 Aponeurosis of gastrocnemius muscle	**11** Medial head of gastrocnemius muscle
3 Extensor digitorum longus muscle	**12** Peroneal artery
4 Extensor hallucis longus muscle	**13** Peroneus brevis muscle
5 Fibula	**14** Peroneus longus muscle
6 Flexor digitorum longus muscle	**15** Posterior tibial artery
7 Flexor hallucis longus muscle	**16** Small saphenous vein
8 Great (long) saphenous vein	**17** Soleus muscle
	18 Tibia
9 Interosseous membrane	**19** Tibialis anterior muscle
	20 Tibialis posterior muscle
	21 Tuberosity of tibia

(a)–(f) Lower leg and ankle, axial MR images.

1 Abductor hallucis muscle	**19** Peroneus tertius muscle
2 Calcaneal tuberosity	**20** Posterior tibial artery and vein
3 Calcaneus	**21** Small saphenous vein
4 Cuboid	**22** Soleus muscle
5 Deltoid ligament	**23** Talus
6 Extensor digitorum muscle	**24** Tendo calcaneus (Achilles' tendon)
7 Extensor hallucis longus muscle	**25** Tendon of extensor digitorum muscle
8 Fibula	**26** Tendon of extensor hallucis longus muscle
9 Flexor accessorius muscle	**27** Tendon of flexor digitorum longus muscle
10 Flexor digitorum longus muscle	**28** Tendon of flexor hallucis longus muscle
11 Flexor hallucis longus muscle	**29** Tendon of peroneus brevis muscle
12 Great (long) saphenous vein	**30** Tendon of peroneus longus muscle
13 Inferior tibiofibular joint	**31** Tendon of plantaris muscle
14 Interosseous membrane	**32** Tendon of tibialis anterior muscle
15 Lateral malleolus	**33** Tendon of tibialis posterior muscle
16 Medial malleolus	**34** Tibia
17 Navicular	**35** Tibialis posterior muscle
18 Peroneus brevis muscle	

(a)–(e) Foot, axial MR images.

1 Abductor digiti minimi muscle
2 Abductor hallucis muscle
3 Calcaneus
4 Deltoid ligament
5 Fibula
6 Flexor accessorius muscle
7 Flexor digitorum brevis muscle
8 Inferior tibiofibular joint
9 Lateral malleolus
10 Medial malleolus
11 Peroneus tertius muscle
12 Plantar aponeurosis
13 Posterior tibial artery
14 Sustentaculum tali
15 Talus
16 Tendon of flexor digitorum longus muscle
17 Tendon of peroneus brevis muscle
18 Tendon of peroneus longus muscle
19 Tendon of tibialis posterior muscle
20 Tibia

(a)–(f) Ankle, sagittal MR images.

1 Abductor digiti minimi muscle	**19** Inferior tibiofibular joint	**37** Superior surface of talus
2 Abductor hallucis muscle	**20** Intermediate cuneiform	**38** Sustentaculum tali
3 Anterior tubercle of calcaneus	**21** Interosseous talocalcaneal ligament	**39** Talonavicular joint
4 Articular cartilage	**22** Lateral cuneiform	**40** Talus
5 Calcaneal tuberosity	**23** Lateral malleolus	**41** Tarsal sinus
6 Calcaneocuboid joint	**24** Medial cuneiform	**42** Tendo calcaneus (Achilles' tendon)
7 Calcaneus	**25** Medial malleolus	**43** Tendon of extensor digitorum muscle
8 Cuboid	**26** Medial subtalar joint	**44** Tendon of extensor hallucis longus muscle
9 Cuneonavicular joint	**27** Navicular	**45** Tendon of flexor digitorum longus muscle
10 Extensor digitorum brevis muscle	**28** Neck of talus	**46** Tendon of flexor hallucis longus muscle
11 Extensor digitorum muscle	**29** Peroneus brevis muscle	**47** Tendon of peroneus brevis muscle
12 Fat pad	**30** Plantar aponeurosis	**48** Tendon of peroneus longus muscle
13 Fibula	**31** Posterior subtalar joint	**49** Tendon of tibialis anterior muscle
14 First metatarsal	**32** Posterior tibial artery and vein	**50** Tendon of tibialis posterior muscle
15 Flexor digitorum brevis muscle	**33** Second metatarsal	**51** Third metatarsal
16 Flexor digitorum longus muscle	**34** Short saphenous vein	**52** Tibia
17 Flexor hallucis longus muscle	**35** Small saphenous vein	**53** Tibiotalar part of ankle joint
18 Head of talus	**36** Soleus muscle	**54** Tuberosity of navicular

Foot, **(a)**–**(e)** oblique axial MR images.
(f)–**(k)** coronal MR images.

1 Abductor digiti minimi muscle	**23** Medial marginal vein
2 Adductor hallucis muscle	**24** Medial plantar nerve and artery
3 Base of metatarsal	**25** Navicular
4 Base of proximal phalanx	**26** Neck of talus
5 Calcaneus	**27** Opponens digiti minimi muscle
6 Cuboid	**28** Plantar aponeurosis
7 Dorsal interossei muscle	**29** Plantar interossei muscle
8 Dorsal venous arch	**30** Shaft of metatarsal
9 Extensor digitorum brevis muscle	**31** Sustentaculum tali
10 Fibula	**32** Talus
11 Flexor accessorius muscle	**33** Tarsal sinus
12 Flexor digiti minimi muscle	**34** Tendon of extensor digitorum longus muscle
13 Flexor digitorum brevis muscle	**35** Tendon of extensor hallucis longus muscle
14 Flexor hallucis brevis muscle	**36** Tendon of flexor digitorum brevis muscle
15 Head of talus	**37** Tendon of flexor digitorum longus muscle
16 Intermediate cuneiform	**38** Tendon of flexor hallucis longus muscle
17 Interossei muscles	**39** Tendon of peroneus brevis muscle
18 Lateral cuneiform	**40** Tendon of peroneus longus muscle
19 Lateral malleolus	**41** Tendon of tibialis anterior muscle
20 Lateral plantar nerve	**42** Tendon of tibialis posterior muscle
21 Medial cuneiform	**43** Tibia
22 Medial malleolus	

Index